Natural Health Peak Performance Longevity Lifestyle

I0101306

By Ralph Teller

Ralph Teller

ISBN-13: 9780615423562

ISBN: 0615423566

First edition

Published by 1Vigor,Inc.

Book covers: Front: Mudford, England. Back: Waterville,
Washington. Both by Ralph Teller

THIS BOOK DOES NOT PROVIDE MEDICAL ADVICE. THE BOOK IS FOR CONSUMER EDUCATIONAL USE ONLY. NOTHING CONTAINED IN THIS BOOK IS OR SHOULD BE CONSIDERED, OR USED AS A SUBSTITUTE FOR, MEDICAL ADVICE, DIAGNOSIS OR TREATMENT. THE BOOK HERE TO EDUCATE CONSUMERS ON HEALTH CARE AND MEDICAL ISSUES THAT MAY AFFECT THEIR DAILY LIVES. THIS BOOK DOE NOT CONSTITUTE THE PRACTICE OF ANY MEDICAL, NURSING OR OTHER PROFESSIONAL HEALTH CARE ADVICE, DIAGNOSIS OR TREATMENT. WE ADVISE READERS TO ALWAYS SEEK THE ADVICE OF A PHYSICIAN OR OTHER QUALIFIED HEALTH CARE PROVIDER WITH ANY QUESTIONS REGARDING PERSONAL HEALTH OR MEDICAL CONDITIONS. NEVER DISREGARD, AVOID OR DELAY IN OBTAINING MEDICAL ADVICE FROM YOUR DOCTOR OR OTHER QUALIFIED HEALTH CARE PROVIDER BECAUSE OF SOMETHING YOU HAVE READ IN THIS BOOK. IF YOU HAVE OR SUSPECT THAT YOU HAVE A MEDICAL PROBLEM OR CONDITION, PLEASE CONTACT A QUALIFIED HEALTH CARE PROFESSIONAL IMMEDIATELY. IF YOU ARE IN THE UNITED STATES AND ARE EXPERIENCING A MEDICAL EMERGENCY, PLEASE CALL 911 OR CALL FOR EMERGENCY MEDICAL HELP ON THE NEAREST TELEPHONE.

INTRODUCTION

This book is about how to naturally achieve optimum health, how to live a high quality and long life, and if an athlete, how to achieve peak performance. The book has a focus on athletic performance because the road to athletic excellence and physical, mental and emotional peak performance is very similar to the path of optimal health and longevity. The lifestyle that leads to a longer, better quality life is the same lifestyle athletes need to follow to reach their ambitions.

There is an art to living. Plato used the expression techne tou biou which means 'the craft of life' which refers to the art of crafting and shaping life. It's an art that has been somewhat lost by our modern culture and modern excesses too focused on immediate gratification, short cuts and quick fixes. The art to optimum health and lifestyle has been lost to the overly busy nature and 'unimportant' distractions of modern life. Modern culture's lifestyle is contributing to high blood pressure, type 2 diabetes, obesity, depression, lack of regular good sleep, chronic fatigue, etc. which underlie many of modern life's sickness and diseases. This book, in part, hopes to impart an appreciation of the need to get back to the basics - the need to live a natural life. The book covers the key ingredients to a long quality life, which include natural nutrition, exercise, strong nerve force and brain power all within a simple lifestyle. I also hope to provide athletes with a larger picture of how they can naturally achieve their athletic goals and mesh those goals with the longer term goals of longevity and long term optimum health.

As maintaining a regular vigorous exercise routine helps us maintain a high and efficient metabolism, to encourage you to engage in the aerobic sports, I provide safety tips and tips on ideal technique for hiking, running, swimming, and cycling.

A key premise of this book is living naturally as the best way to achieve optimum health, longevity and peak performance. As such, I provide natural tips on (i) the benefits of natural nutrition and portion control, (ii) the benefits of obtaining sufficient Vitamin D levels from the sun, (iii) how to obtain natural regular good sleep, (iv) how to naturally beat depression, and (v) how to naturally quit smoking cigarettes. As maintaining high testosterone levels is important to men's health and vitality, we recommend natural ways to increase testosterone levels. The book also recommends natural ways to increase the production of the growth hormones essential to growth and healing. Since women have unique health considerations, the book provides insight into the the role of Calcium and Iron in women's health and provides natural food sources of obtaining both nutrients.

For athletes I recommend natural ways to maintain kidney health, as the kidneys play a key role in the production of red blood cells, essential to oxygen delivery to our cells for peak athletic performance. Maintaining healthy kidneys is also important to everyone in fighting fatigue. There is a list of natural food sources that provide the key nutrients needed to produce red blood cells. While not advocating caffeine, it is recognized caffeine can play a role in certain athletic and other endeavors, the book provides caffeine strategies.

As maintaining strong nerves and efficient management of our metabolism is essential to optimal health and life quality, I provide natural solutions to building strong nerve force through proper breathing rhythm and lowering of our resting heart rate.

Recognizing the importance of the mental and emotional aspects of peak performance and the Ideal Performance State necessary for reaching optimum athletic and other potentials, we provide insight into the Ideal Performance State. There is a section on mental toughness and a section on how mental imagery skills can be developed to give each of us an edge in our challenges.

Keeping our minds sharp and brains healthy is essential to our life quality and longevity. I provide natural tips and insight into (i) creativity skills, (ii) clear thinking skills, (iii) the importance of heightened sense and expanded awareness, and (iv) self-actualization skills.

Lifestyle plays a key role in our life quality and lifespan. The book suggests a more simple lifestyle as a way to care for our soul and nourish our spirit and offer tips on how this can be accomplished. By simple, I do not imply boring, dull or unaccomplished. I also touch base on how developing leadership skills can play an important role in life quality.

DEDICATION

This book is dedicated to my parents Ralph Howard Teller and Helen Teller of Long Island, New York who have lived hard working, quiet, unpretentious, and simple lives of integrity. This book is also dedicated to my two children, Luke Teller and Danielle Teller, who provide inspiration in their bold and successful opening of their unique Afterlife Boutique, a vintage clothing store in the Mission District of San Francisco, during difficult economic times. This book is also dedicated to my aunt Gloria Tarsy of Long Island, New York who pointed me in the right direction during my youth and continuously shares her wisdom. This book is inspired by Chris Harig of Issaquah, Washington, who at 37 become the 2010 USA Long Course Duathlon National Champion, while raising his young family and maintaining his responsibilities at Microsoft. Chris represents the quiet unflamboyant bedrock of American prosperity. This book is also inspired by Gerry Marvin of Seattle, Washington whose upbeat tenacity and discipline triumphed from injuries sustained in a 2007 serious bike accident to a phenomenal performance at the 2010 Ironman Canada Triathlon that earned him a slot at the 2010 Ironman World Championship in Kona.

CONTENTS

ACKNOWLEDGMENTS

I'd like to thank the contributing writers (experts in topics relating to natural health, peak performance and longevity) that help make www.1vigor.com successful, including Chris Harig of Issaquah, Washington (Running); Valerie Pierce of Dublin, Ireland (Clear Thinking Skills); Dan Ballbach of Seattle, Washington (Leadership); Christina Geithner of Spokane, Washington (Yoga); Paul Bennett, Jr. of Saratoga Springs, New York (Nutrition); James Styler of Christ Church, New Zealand (Endurance Running); Jessica Ippoliti of Corte Madera, California (Sports Massage); and Michelle Simmons of Kaneohe, Hawaii (Open Water Swimming).

1 LONGEVITY LIFESTYLE

Commit to a Longevity Lifestyle. Naturally achieving wellness, longevity and living a vigorous fuller life is a commitment to a lifestyle that combines, like finely woven fabric, (i) a diet of natural nutrition, (ii) regular exercise routine, (iii) strong nerve force achieved with good and regularly scheduled sleep, meditation and proper breathing, and (iv) a philosophy that embraces determination and discipline, responsibility and challenge, positive relationships and productive endeavors, and clear thinking and simple living.

Wellness and longevity is achieved in part by developing, maintaining and managing a high and efficient metabolism. Various cultures can offer different perspectives and insights into the longevity lifestyle. Although not examining longevity in terms of metabolism, the Eastern philosophy of Tao, which means 'Way' or path, teaches that one can reach the state of being of 'Enlightenment' and a long life by living in harmony with the ebb and flow forces of nature. (I interpet this, in part, to equate to metabolism management.) This enlightenment is achieved through the greatest of personal effort and self-discipline. Taoism equates physical and mental health and provides that only a strong and healthy body can house a strong and healthy spirit. It's a holistic approach to health and spiritual advancement. Taoism believes human life is comprised of 'Three Treasures': Essense (jing), Energy (chee) and Spirit (shen). These three fundamental and interdependent levels of being, the physical, energetic and mental are the natural legacy of life. It is their relative strength and balance and our level of discipline in 'guarding' these treasures that determines our longevity and level of health and wellness.

Similarly, each of us has the opportunity, if we live well, to achieve the same or better level of health and vigor tomorrow as we have today. That philosophy adhered to and practiced each day over the years can add many years to life expectancy. Good years! Advances in science and technologies hold the promise to extend a high quality life even further.

Each of us also has the potential to live essentially free from illness and disease and when illness strikes it will be short, mild and not become a setback.

A day filled with nutrition, exercise, proper breathing, challenge, focused positive thinking and rest is accretive and builds the foundation for stronger brain power, a stronger immune system and nerve force cumulatively for more vital stronger living.

Efficiency and Metabolism.   Eastern philosophy also instructs that each of us are conceived with a certain amount of primordial energy (yuan-chee). This primordial energy can be compared to the potential energy stored in a battery. This primordial energy begins to dissipate at birth and the rate of dissipation determines one's lifespan. Our batteries are charged, the rate of energy dissipation is slowed and life is prolonged by eating nutritiously and breathing correctly. This thinking seems wise and correlates back to metabolism management.

A key element in building longevity is to reach a point of optimum metabolic efficiency. This is achieved through (i) a diet rich in nutrition, (ii) long and deep breathing which increases the supply of air and oxygen with less effort, (iii) achieving and maintaining an optimal body weight which lowers the overhead required for the best functioning of the vital organs and muscles, and lowers stress on our joints, (iv) exercise, which builds and maintains a strong metabolism and (v) clear and positive thinking. Our metabolism can be efficiently focused to elongate our life through good and strong living. Metabolic efficiency is achieved at the cellular, organ and system levels. The more efficient and strong our metabolism, the longer and stronger our life will be.

Natural Nutrition. It is recommended that (i) 3/5 of your natural diet should consist of natural fruits and vegetables, (ii) 1/5 of your diet should be sources of protein such as organic meat, chicken, fish, eggs, nuts, beans and lentils, and (iii) 1/5 of our diet come from natural oils such as olive oil or peanuts, and natural sweets and starches, such as molasses and potatoes, respectively. Natural food like whole grains, vegetables and fruits that directly capture the sun's energy are rich in Vitamin B complex and other vitamins, proteins, minerals and carbohydrates. Most processed foods are devitalized of nutrients. Historically whole grains have sustained flourishing civilizations beginning with the grains cultivated in the rich river valleys of Mesopotamia. Whole grains like wheat, oats, rice, corn, barley, rye, spelt make easy to prepare cereals and contain nutrients far in excess of the commercially processed cereals.

Dairy products like cheese, cottage cheese and yogurt are excellent sources of calcium, protein, carbohydrates, Vitamin D, and electrolytes (sodium and potassium). Plain yogurt has a sweetness in and of itself and does not need added sweetening. It's interesting to note that Dutch men have become the tallest men on the planet. Dairy products are the primary food staple in the Netherlands and the increased height of Dutch men have been attributed in part to their rich consumption of dairy products.

Incidently, eating nutritious natural foods is mostly less expensive than eating processed foods.

Hydration and Milk. Good and ample hydration is essential for everybody, but particularly for very active individuals and competitive athletes. Milk is an excellent primary source of hydration as it is an excellent source of calcium, protein, carbohydrates and Vitamin D and also contains just the right percentage of potassium and sodium that supports maximum nutrient absorption and helps maintain ideal salt balances. Nonfat milk or low fat milk is preferred in the warm climates and during summer. Low fat milk or whole milk is better in the winter as the extra natural fats help generate heat internally to stay warm. Milk is a better source of hydration and is also good food. Reliance on water alone for hydration can have the effect of flushing needed vitamins and minerals from the body.

Good Breathing Technique. We've all experienced the fast pulse and faster breathing that comes with anticipation of an important event, like giving a speech. Advice typically given is to 'take a deep breath and relax'. That's exactly right! Deep, slow, quiet and regular long breathing is relaxing to our system and is the correct way to breath. Breathing should be long and deep where the abdomen (not just the chest) expands with each inhalation. Deep abdominal breathing (i) increases the supply of oxygen into the blood stream as more air moves into the lower and larger sections of the lungs, (ii) helps better peristalsis necessary for optimal intestinal digestion, (iii) stimulates blood circulation in the abdominal cavity, (iv) encourages deep uninterrupted sleep, (v) calms emotions and (vi) sharpens awareness. Correct breathing also means inhaling through the nose. The nose and naval cavity play the essential role of (i) warming or cooling the air to within 1 degree of body temperature, (ii) humidifying the air and (iii) filtering dust and other particles.

Regular Vigorous Exercise. Exercise enhances and increases blood flow to each cell and to the vital organs bringing more oxygen and more nutrients to both and improving the cell performance and organ function. Exercise strengthens metabolism, extends our life's 'battery' and builds cell, organ and metabolic efficiency. Learning a sport builds confidence. Exercise makes us happy. The best form of exercise is aerobic exercise. Five days a week we should engage in at least one hour of vigorous exercise. Hiking, Swimming, Cycling and Running are excellent forms of aerobic exercise. An exercise routine that combines all four is ideal. On average, beginning at age 25, our lung capacity decreases by 1% per year. Swimming slows down this shrinkage and can increase lung capacity.

Simple Lifestyle and Productive Endeavors. Days are best filled with meeting personal responsibilities, challenge and productive endeavors where there is an opportunity to learn, teach, contribute and improve skills. Adversity and challenge builds character and sharpens focus. The belief that the easy life is a good life is an illusion as a soft life is most often a weak life. The good life is a strong life. Worry and unexpected hardships occur in the ordinary course and play a maturing role. However, extreme worry destroys health, damages the immune system and weakens the cardiovascular and nervous system. A simple life, and that does not mean a dull or boring life, is a life of lower and better managed worries. A simple life can be a life of significant accomplishment, achievement and reward.

Strong Nerve Force and Good Natural Sleep. A simple but full life is a key ingredient to longevity. Good regular sleep is essential to optimum long term health. Good sleep is earned. Hard work followed by good sleep, like the yin and yang, the day and the night, and the changing seasons is the natural rhythm of life. An average of regularly scheduled 8 hours of sleep each day is essential to a high quality life. During deep sleep (i) blood pressure drops, breathing slows and muscles relax which gives the nervous system an opportunity to rest, (ii) growth and other hormones are released into the blood stream, (iii) blood supply to the muscles increases and (iv) tissue growth, development and repair occurs, including muscle growth and repair, and energy is restored. Rapid Eye Movement sleep (REM sleep), which accounts for 25% of our sleep, provides energy to the brain and the body. Living a life of integrity, self respect and respect of others helps sleep with a clear conscience and is a very important factor in getting a good night's sleep.

2 EXERCISE

Health Benefits of Aerobic Sports and Activities. The are significant health benefits in participating in aerobic sports such as cycling, hiking, walking, swimming, running. These benefits include (i) improved metabolism efficiency, (ii) increased nutrients to cells and organs due to increased blood circulation to all parts of the body, (iii) restorative health due to a stronger immune system, (iv) improved quality and longevity of life, (v) better sex and (vi) a feeling of lasting wellness.

Engaging in sports has other tremendous benefits. In addition to improving physical health, sports offer the opportunity to learn new skills, teach, build mental toughness, sharpen focus and clear thinking skills, compete, learn team and Leadership skills, learn from failures, build confidence and make friends.

Everyone, children, young adults and adults, should be encouraged to engage in sports. All sports are good, but it is the aerobic sports which are most physically beneficial.

Recent studies have found that vigorous physical activity is even more protective than moderate activity, provided it is not overdone. Regular vigorous aerobic activity improves aerobic fitness reducing hypertension risks. Furthermore, a recent study has found that the risks of hypertension and high blood pressure are significantly reduced when aerobic fitness activities where at their highest. Hypertension can be avoided if people improve their fitness. Regular vigorous aerobic activity is the principal behavioral determinant of fitness, and that being more physically active can improve one's fitness. But the activity needs to be moderate to vigorous to adequately improve fitness to see the greater health benefits.

Regular physical aerobic activity should be encouraged in young adulthoods because activity behaviors tend to track over time. Activity and fitness count in relation to the long-term prevention or development of heart disease. We can adopt good habits early on! However, we are all encouraged to develop a balanced aerobic exercise routine!

Too little competition or challenge or too much overstimulation or stress reduces our ability to effectively cope with the challenges of competition and life! As exercise provides a good outlet for competition and challenge, we are encouraging you to engage in at least one of the aerobic exercise of walking, hiking, running, swimming or cycling. For each of these activities we provide you with how to engage in each of the activities safely. You will also find tips on good technique for swimming, running and cycling.

Walking, Hiking and The Outdoors

"When man knows how to live dangerously, he is not afraid to die. When he is not afraid to die, he is, strangely, free to live. When he is free to live, he can become bold, courageous, reliant." William O. Douglas, Of Men and Mountains.

For the adventure of a lifetime, the team of Lewis and Clark set out from the Missouri Territory in 1804 to explore the West, discover new plant and wildlife and find a waterway passageway to the Pacific. We can all capture a slice of this adventure and exploration by hiking our plains, prairies, deserts, woods, forests, mountains, rivers and coasts.

Hiking and being in The Outdoors improves metabolism efficiency, brings nutrients to cells due to increased blood circulation to all parts of the body, refreshes attitude and promotes lasting wellness. Hiking and being in The Outdoors makes for a better quality and fuller life and enhances Longevity.

The Ten Essentials for Every Hiking Trip:

Navigation (map and compass)
Sun protection
Insulation (extra clothing)
Illumination (flashlight/headlamp)
First-aid supplies
Fire
Repair kit and tools
Nutrition (extra food)
Hydration (extra water)
Emergency shelter

Keep a Log of your hiking adventures!

There is simple and exhilarating joy, freedom and adventure in being in the forests, mountains, wilderness, seas, rivers, plains and deserts. John Muir wrote "Walk quietly in any direction and taste the freedom of the mountaineer." This unique sense of freedom is achievable in The Outdoors. Break away from modern day conveniences and become a part of The Outdoors for good physical and mental health.

Mountaineering offers many challenges and skills and requires continual awareness of the (i) situation and environment at hand, (ii) weather, (iii) terrain, (iv) focus required on balance and the simple tasks of hand and foot placement when life is placed in risk, (v) right equipment and its limitations, (vi) individual and team strengths and shortcomings, (vii) needed problem solving skills and good judgment, (viii) service to protecting wilderness (leave no trace), and (ix) physical and mental preparation.

Health Benefits of Swimming. Swim for Longevity. Swimming is the most beneficial of the aerobic sports because it increases lung capacity, utilizes many muscles in the body, is great for energizing the vital organs, and is very low impact. Swimming builds metabolic efficiency and is a good exercise in breathing control. Swimming also makes the heart bigger and stronger.

Studies have shown that Swimmers have higher Lung volumes and capacities than land based athletes and non athletes. Swim training studies have also demonstrated increases in total lung capacities and vital capacity in children and young adults. This is believed so because (i) swimmers breath against the resistance of water in a restricted breathing pattern with repeated expansion of the lungs and (ii) swimming takes place with the body in a horizontal position and this posture is optimal for perfusion of the lung capacity and diffusion of respiratory gases.

Water can have a soothing calming emotional effect. Swimming in a pool, lake or ocean can be like a mini vacation. Swimming extends life! There is beauty and art in developing a good swim stroke. Mastering this sport by developing a sleek stroke is an excellent challenge and discipline.

Freestyle Swimming Technique. It is estimated that 70% of your swim speed comes from stroke mechanics and only 30% from the muscles. Swim technique for freestyle swimming, the most popular of the four main swim strokes, can vary somewhat depending upon whether you are a short course, long course or open water distance swimmer. Total Immersion, by Terry Laughlin is an excellent book for learning a relaxed and streamlined stroke technique, perhaps geared more toward long course and open water swimming than short course sprinters. Good Ironman 70.3 or full Ironman Triathlon swimming technique incorporates many of the swim tips below.

However regardless of whether you swim short or long course, or open water, good swimming technique seeks to achieve the following:

- Streamlined body with legs and torso high in the water to lessen drag.

- Chest leaning downward or 'Pressing the Buoy'. This action tends to lift the legs upward into a streamlined position.

- Long forward stretch of the arm that reaches and extends your length by several inches.

- Early catch of the water with a high elbow focused on propelling the body forward that creates your hand and your forearm (not just your hand) as your paddle. A high early elbow bend helps set up the early catch and using both the hand and forearm.

- Accelerate your hand during the second half of each stroke. Watch your traction as you anchor and pull with your hand and forearm. If your hands are going faster than your body is moving in the water, your hand and forearm are slipping and not gripping the water. This is probably due to a low elbow position or slipping arm.

- Long follow through on the down stroke to get the maximum propulsion from a each stroke. Dropping the shoulder at the very end of the stroke lengthens the stroke a few inches.

- Streamlined kick that stays within the body's shadow so as to not create a drag. This is accomplished by relying more on the hips to start the kick and less on knee flexion. Toes should be pointed to minimize drag.

- Head streamlined with the body that turns to the side instead of upward or forward when breathing, as lifting the head up tends to lead the body out of a streamlined position.

- Body roll from stroke to stroke that lessens drag and is the initial power behind each stroke. The longer you stay on your side in each stroke cycle the faster and farther your body will travel. This roll rhythm movement starts in the body's center or core and uses the hips. It is recommended to lead each stroke with the hips.

- Take deep satisfying breaths and exhale under water.

Long course swimmers are encouraged to learn 'front quadrant' swim technique which recommends beginning each down stroke after the recovering arm has past the head.

Cycling

"Everybody wants to know what I'm on. What am I on? I'm on my bike busting my ass six hours a day. What are you on? " - Lance Armstrong

Two wheels can make you memories of a lifetime! Cycling can be road, off-road, mountain and touring, all of which offer great health and challenge, in addition to adventure and good scenery! It's easy to find local teams of your skill level to ride with and local bike shops to help you find the right bike for your needs. Learn how cycling technique and safety, improved pedaling mechanics, good cycling hydration and injury prevention improve cycling skills and performance and help to achieve greater health, better muscle tone, enhanced Longevity, and a more energetic and fuller life.

Cycling Technique and Pedaling Mechanics

- Learn not to "mash" gears and instead learn how to achieve a higher cadence (RPMs) will allow you to cycle and race faster and more efficiently.
- Pedaling should be envisioned as pedaling more in "circles". Although some research suggests that a combination of pedaling in circles with a little more juice (mashing) on the down stroke.
- During the recovery period of a pedal stroke, continue the circular motion of pedaling, while pulling up on the

pedal at the same time. A common mistakes in cycling is only pushing down on the pedals and not pulling up. By just mashing, you are losing the power potential of the upstroke. Maximum power is achieved in a 360 degree stroke effort.

- Avoid rocking motion while cycling.
- Avoid bouncing while cycling.
- Keep your upper body motionless. Avoid allowing your hips to rock from side to side. An upper motionless body helps maintain energy focused on moving the bike straight forward. You will get more force to the pedals and more forward momentum if you can become fluid in getting the power from the pedal stroke to your legs.
- Higher Cadences: Cadence is defined in RPM's. An RPM's between 90-110 is considered ideal. This is definitely a learned skill. Riding in the smaller gear is the best way to improve RPM's. It is recommend the first 40 minutes of a ride be done in the smaller gear at a higher cadence. The use of higher cadences produces more efficient cycling, with less fatigue to your legs because you will be using less Type 2 muscle fibers (fast twitch muscles) that fatigue more easily. By minimizing the use of your fast twitch fibers you will: (i) decrease glycogen use (burn less fuel), (ii) decrease lactate production (which is when you start to feel the burning sensation during the workout),and (iii) as a result, you will experience less muscle fatigue.

11 Cycling Safety Tips

- Obey Traffic Laws.
- Familiarize yourself with all applicable traffic laws and cycling rules. Do not run stop signs or red lights or use the wrong side of the street. Be respectful.
- Ride on Same Side of Traffic. It is generally either illegal or unsafe to ride on a sidewalk or on the road towards

oncoming traffic. Join In. If you are traveling at the same speed as other traffic, it may be safer to jump in and ride with traffic and be more visible to motorists.

- Wear Your Helmet. Always wear a helmet and make sure it is properly fastened and fitted.

- Make Eye Contact with Driver. Making eye contact with drivers ensures that the motorists see you and helps you assert your rightful place on the road.

- Ride Straight and Consistent. Do not weave in and out of traffic. Ride consistently and predictably. Inconsistent conduct increases your chances of being squeezed out of traffic or getting hit.

- Ride Defensively. Make sure you are always aware of your surroundings. Know what is behind you and watch out for what is in front of you. Be on the lookout for road hazards, sand and gravel, glass, railroad tracks, parked cars, snow and slush. Sewer grates and cracks in the road can catch your wheel. Watch for parked cars where people may be opening.

- Wear Bright Clothing. Have reflectors on front, side and rear of bike and wear bright clothing.

- Use Your Hands. Always keep at least one hand on the handle bars and use your hands to signal turns and lane changes.

- Maintain Brakes. Keep breaks in good condition and be aware of how weather can affect braking ability.

- Keep Ears Attentive. Keep your ears attentive. Don't ride with an iPod or cover your ears with clothing.

*The first 10 tips are courtesy of David Zabriskie's Yield to Life.

Running. Running offers so much more than a better muscle tone and a longer and more energetic life. For many, body and soul tune into this invigorating activity. Running can be a great adventure from the routine and an opportunity to escape or clear one's mind. So what are you waiting for? The sooner you get started the better! There are lots of great books and publications on good running shoes and clothing, proper nutrition and hydration, and how to prevent injury.

Good Running Technique

- Foot plant is primarily on the balls and mid section of the foot reducing bone impact and breaking forces while strengthening the lower leg tendons, joints and muscles.
- Foot strikes the ground a few inches in front of the center of gravity. Note that over striding causes excessive braking. The key is pushing into the ground and exerting a lot of energy off the ground with the shortest amount of ground contact time. The fastest runners spend the least time with their foot on the ground. The objective is to maximize force into the ground, but get off quickly.
- Drive off ground with your toes.
- Maximize stride length by using the hip flexors to lift the knee up and forward.
- Keep head upright and looking straight ahead.
- Shoulders and upper body are kept totally relaxed to conserve energy and provide balance.
- Keep shoulders down and back.
- Develop a strong core. Building a strong core is key for many sports and activities.
- Elbow retains close to a 90 angle and never comes further forward than the abdominal area.
- Arms never cross mid section to avoid unnecessary side to side motion.
- Do not tightly clench fist. This conserves energy and lessens tension.
- Keep the swing leg near parallel to the ground and avoid reaching too high to the buttock.
- Keep the back and body's mid section erect. Keep the entire body in line from the ankles to the ears.

- Maintain a slight lean forward through the entire body to provide momentum and conserve energy. This slight tilt should start at the ankles and not at the hips.

Running Hydration. Good Hydration is essential to maintain peak performance for very active individuals and competitive athletes, especially Runners. However, reliance on water alone for hydration, or excess water consumption, can have the effect of flushing needed vitamins and minerals from the body. The more active one is the greater one's hydration needs. Hydration is important for runner particularly when running long distances. Hydration is equally as important during cold weather as it is in hot, dry or humid weather. In cold weather, dehydration can cause hypothermia very quickly. Drinking plenty of fluids during cold weather is essential to maintain core body temperatures.

When running in hot weather, the combination of the external heat and the internal heat produced from running, heat within the body can build causing Hyperthermia which is having a core body temperature that is too high. Maintaining good hydration can reduce the onset of Hyperthermia as good hydration enhances sweating which acts to cool core body temperatures.

In very humid weather, our sweat doesn't evaporate as very well and we tend to sweat more with less cooling effect thereby loosing needed fluids to maintain good performance. When lost fluids are not replaced our body begins to shut down starting with heat cramps and muscle cramps due to lack of electrolytes. Fatigue will begin to increase when fluids are not replaced and under extreme lack of fluid replacement heat exhaustion or stroke can occur.

It is recommended we drink between 14 and 27 ounces of fluid each hour running. It is also recommended to maintain best performance that fluids contain electrolytes, carbohydrates, calcium and protein. Interestingly, Nonfat Milk contains a natural mix of electrolytes (Yes, milk is high in Potassium!), carbohydrates and protein and is a good source of Hydration when the weather is cooler or in early morning rides.

3 NATURAL NUTRITION

Natural Nutrition and Portion Control. Eating natural foods and eating only the amount of calories our bodies need to be strong and fit is part of a greater lifestyle choice and philosophy. A healthier lifestyle philosophy is to live prudently and efficiently, consuming only what we need. Many of our modern lifestyle diseases, such obesity, hypertension and heart disease are the result of eating heavily processed foods, more calories than our bodies need and consuming excess salt and trans fats and hydrogenated oils. Our food habits also impact our resting heart rate - an important health indicator.

Numerous studies (with yeast and mammals) clearly indicated that longevity is significantly enhanced with a calorie restrictive diet. In these studies it is possible this enhanced life span is in part due to adaptation ability that maximizes utilization of the lower calories creating some metabolic efficiency. These studies also support the conclusion that the quality of the restricted calories can be as important a factor as portion control.

There is a relatively new theory that low-calorie diets activate genes designed to help animals endure hard times, which boost cellular repair mechanisms. There is evidence that almost all animals, including humans, may have a similar suite of genes.

The challenge for each of us is to find the right mix of calorie count with the best calorie quality to reach our optimum body weight that sustains a high but efficient metabolism. Calorie intake needs to support and maintain a high metabolism that supports an active lifestyle and routine that includes vigorous exercise. Portion control should not sacrifice a high metabolism as the objective is not to live a longer but weaker and restrictive life, but to instead lead a longer, stronger and more vital life. Olympic swimmer Michael Phelps consumes 10,000 calories to support his ideal metabolism needs.

The quality of our calories is very important. A high quality nutritious diet helps us achieve metabolic efficiency. The highest nutritional food is that produced naturally and organically. Fruits, vegetables, and whole grains are packed with nutrients. Processed food is devitalized of essential vitamins, minerals and energy and is filled with empty calories. Natural food has been produced capturing the energy of the sun. In many instances, organically grown food has a higher nutrition content than artificially fertilized mass produced foods. As most European farms are smaller than the large American farms, European farmers are able to build and maintain rich soils by fertilizing their land with manure (mostly cow) instead of artificial and incomplete fertilizers used by large American farmers. Rich soils produce a higher crop yield with a higher nutrient content. American organic farming attempts to follow the European experience.

Health Benefits of Vitamin D. Vitamin D is one of the body's most essential nutrients as it (i) plays a key role in the absorption of calcium for the maintenance of health bones, (ii) promotes muscle development and muscle strength, (iii) appears to play a role in cardiovascular health, metabolic health, immune system strength and cancer prevention, and (iv) plays a positive role in mental health and depression avoidance. As Vitamin D receptors have been discovered in most cells of the body, expanded research on other health benefits of Vitamin D are being examined. The role of Vitamin D in health and disease is continually expanding. On the other hand, excessive exposure to the sun has been proven to cause certain types of skin cancer later in life. The purpose of this article is to educate you on the essential health benefits and process of Vitamin D production initiated from the Sun and the risks of sun induced skin damage and cancer.

Skin Vitamin D Synthesis from the Sun, Food Sources of Vitamin D. There are 3 sources of Vitamin D:

1. The SUN! The major source of Vitamin D for most humans is from the skin's exposure to the ultraviolet B (UVB) rays of sunlight. Sunlight contributes on average over 90% of our Vitamin D!

2. Food Sources. Only a few food sources naturally contain appreciable sources of Vitamin D3 that have an impact on dietary intake: fish, fish liver, fish liver oils, fatty fish, mushrooms, egg yolks and beef liver. Mushrooms are the only vegan source of Vitamin D. Fish liver oils, such as cod liver oil, appear to have the greatest concentration of Vitamin D containing 1 Tbs. (15 ml) provides 1360 IU (90.6 IU/ml). Fish should be consumed that live only in uncontaminated waters.

Oily fish such as catfish, salmon, sardine, tuna, mackerel and blue fish are excellent sources of Vitamin D3. A serving of wild salmon can have up to 1000 IU of Vitamin D3. NOTE, farm raised salmon have only about 1/4 the amount of Vitamin D as wild salmon. The disparity of Vitamin D content between farm raised salmon and wild salmon is very interesting. Assuming all other things being equal, farm raised salmon don't have the natural survival challenges (ie. currents, swimming long distances, swimming upstream, spawning, chasing food, eluding predators such as Orca whales, seals and sea lions) as do wild salmon. Are wild salmon more vital and stronger than farm salmon? Undoubtedly! By way of analogy are people more physically active more vital than sedate inactive people? Do more physically active people have higher demands for Vitamin D?

Some countries practice fortification of certain foods with Vitamin D3, most often milk, yogurt, butter and cheese. Orange juice is also sometimes fortified with Vitamin D3.

3. Vitamin D Supplements. Vitamin D supplements in different dosages are widely and inexpensively available in most countries. While with any supplement there is a concern about toxicity, studies thus far have indicated Vitamin D supplements are safe.

Vitamin D Synthesis and Metabolism. Our body's absorption of energy from sun to create Vitamin D is one of the many wonders of the human body. It's a complex process, but an important process to appreciate for people tuned into optimum health and peak performance, like athletes.

Our body's absorption of energy (photons) from the sun to create Vitamin D may be as significant to animal life (all animals generate Vitamin D from the sun) as the process of photosynthesis is necessary for plant life. The process of plant photosynthesis also uses the energy from the sun to convert carbon dioxide and water into organic compounds, especially sugars. In photosynthesis, plants release oxygen as a waste product. As well as maintaining the normal level of oxygen in the atmosphere, nearly all life either depends on photosynthesis directly as a source of energy, or indirectly as the ultimate source of the energy in their food.

The body's process of making Vitamin D begins in the skin. The skin contains 7-dehydrocholesterol (7-DHC), which is a derivative of cholesterol. 7-DHC absorbs photons from UVB rays of the sun that occur within the 280-320 nm wave length. This synthesis creates pre-Vitamin D. Vitamin D metabolism then occurs in the liver where it is stored until it is needed. However, from the liver, Vitamin D then passes through the kidneys. Following the final converting step in the kidneys the physiologically active form of vitamin D is released into the blood for circulation.

Factors Impacting Skin Vitamin D Synthesis. As the skin's exposure to the sun's ultraviolet B radiation is our bodies major source of Vitamin D, it is important to know and understand the various factors that impact this Vitamin D synthesis caused by the sun.

Here are key factors impacting skin Vitamin D synthesis:

1. Content of 7-dehydrocholesterol (7-DHC) in the Skin. 7-DHC content in the skin is a primary factor in the occurance of Vitamin D synthesis.

2. UVB Wavelength. Vitamin D synthesis occurs primarily in the UVB wavelength between 280 nm and 320 nm which impacts the energy of the photons which cause Vitamin D synthesis.

3. Solar Zenith Angle, a function of Latitude, Season and Time of Day. Before solar UVB can intiate Vitamin D synthesis in the skin it must traverse the atmosphere. The main determinant of available UVB is the angle of the sun. The more directly overhead the position of the sun the more UVB is available to for Vitamin D synthesis. Latitude, season and time of day are the three factors impacting available UVB. The higher the latitude, the closer to winter season and the further from mid day, the less UVB is available for Vitamin D synthesis. Conversly, the the closer to the equater, the summer season and mid day, the more UVB is available. The more UVB available, the less time in the sun is needed to meet Vitamin D needs from synthesis.

For instance, at the latitude of Seattle, Boston, München, Hobart and Christchurch, Vitamin D synthesis occurs between about 7am to 5pm during summer. In the spring and fall, the window for Vitamin D synthesis shortens to about 9am to 3pm. In winter the window for Vitamin D synthesis decreased altogether. In summer, morning is a good time to get sun for Vitamin D production with low risk for UV skin damage.

4. Altitude. As higher altitudes result in shorter distances and less atmosphere for UVB to pass through, more UVB is available to reach the skin for Vitamin D synthesis. The amount of available

UVB increases by 4% for every 300 meters (984 feet) of elevation gain.

5. Atmospheric Conditions. Cloud cover is a very important factor determining UVB available for Vitamin D synthesis. Lower thicker clouds have the greatest ability to decrease available UVB. Heavy cloud cover can block 99% of UVB from reaching the ground.

Airborne pollutants can significantly reduce available UVB. Tall city buildings, narrow city streets, along with the move to indoor jobs would have certainly decreased sun exposure amongst urban populations.

Snow can reflect 90% of UV radiation greatly increasing the available UVB striking the skin.

6. Skin Tone, Pigmentation. Studies show lighter skin tones have greater capacity to synthesize Vitamin D and require less UVB exposure to produce adequate levels of Vitamin D. While people in the United States in general have become increasingly Vitamin D deficient with almost half of the population Vitamin D deficient, researchers have found that more than half of African Americans were Vitamin D deficient. Darkly pigmented skin isn't as efficient at inducing Vitamin D synthesis. This is not a problem in Africa where there is plenty of sun, but often translates into Vitamin D deficiency in more northern latitudes where sunshine is more limited.

7. Body Mass Index (BMI). Research confirms people with a BMI >30 has an effect on Vitamin D levels as obese people generally have lower levels of Vitamin D and a slightly reduced rated of UVB induced production of Vitamin D.

8. Age. The capacity for Vitamin D synthesis is based upon the availability of 7-DHC in the skin. Aging generally reduces the content of 7-DHC in the skin and thus the potential for Vitamin

D production. The 7-DHC skin content seems to reduce by about one half between the age of 20 and 90. Vitamin D supplements, a diet rich in Vitamin D and increased sun exposure, but not excessive sun exposure, is recommended with aging.

9. Sun Avoidance, Sunscreen and Clothing. It's been estimated that the correct application of sunscreen, which blocks UVB rays, with an SPF of 8 reduces the skins Vitamin D production by over 90% and sunscreen with an SPF of 15 reduces Vitamin D production by 99%. Sun avoidance (as in staying indoors) and clothing and hats can significantly reduce sun induced Vitamin D production.

Risks of Vitamin D Deficiency. Vitamin D deficiency carries the following health risks:

1. Poor Bone and Muscle Health. As Vitamin D plays an essential role to calcium absorption, weak bones and muscle can occur when Vitamin D is deficient. Calcium and Vitamin K are also essential to bone health. See Natural Sources of Calcium. See also Natural Sources of Vitamin K.

2. Multiple Sclerosis. Research indicates the people who are Vitamin D deficient at an early age are at greater risk of developing multiple sclerosis in later years of life. Some studies have strongly indicated that pre-natal Vitamin D is an key risk factor for developing multiple. sclerosis later in life. There is a greater risk of multiple sclerosis living in northern latitudes compared to living near the equator. Women who supplement their diet with Vitamin D are proven to have a lower risk of multiple sclerosis.

3. Depression. Sunshine and Vitamin D levels have been proven to positively impact mental health and help fight and prevent depression. See Tips to Beat Depression Naturally

4. Cancer Prevention. As part of the paradox between DNA skin damage due to sun overexposure, and the health benefits of Vitamin D, researchers have found that chronic sun exposure (and hence consistently high levels of Vitamin D) confers protection against Melanoma. High Vitamin D levels are also now believed to play a role to protect against stomach, colorectum, liver, gallbladder, pancreas, lung, breast, prostate, bladder and kidney cancers. Although sun exposure may confer protective effect for melanoma and many other cancers, it simultaneously promotes squamous cell and and basal cell carcinoma.

5. Tuberculosis. Sunshine and Vitamin D have been proven to help fight and cure tuberculosis.

Sun Overexposure, Photoprotection and Healthy Skin. The effects of sun exposure are paradoxical with (i) skin cell DNA damage risk increasing with excessive sun exposure over decades on the one hand, and (ii) the essential health needs of Vitamin D synthesis from sun exposure on the other. In fair skinned individuals, maximum possible Vitamin D synthesis can occur within a few minutes of mid day summer sun exposure. Yet, Over the course of two decades, Vitamin D levels have dramatically decreased among Americans. Since sunlight is the body's major source of Vitamin D, increases in sunscreen, sun avoidance, and overall decreased outdoor activity, while successful in reducing skin cancers, has probably reduced vitamin D levels in the population.

Recommended Dosage of Sun Exposure. Implementing guidelines suggesting sun exposure duration for sufficient Vitamin D3 production is difficult due to the the complex and various factors that impact Vitamin D synthesis. As such, the medical profession believes at this point that no recommendation on sun exposure can be made that is both safe and accurate enough for general public usage. It seems many in the medical profession consider the risk of skin cancer from unprotected sun exposure outweighs any increase Vitamin D levels that may occur, and recommend Vitamin D supplements.

Sun Overexposure and Skin Aging. Excessive sun exposure over years can prematurely age skin. Eye Health. UV rays can also cause damage to the eyes. Sunglasses can protect eyes from sun damage. The ideal pair of sunglasses would block all UV rays while not sacrificing the transmission of visible light.

Hydration and Electrolyte Balance. Maintaining Hydration and Electrolyte Balance is critical to nerve and muscle function, and as such, is a key consideration for athletes hoping to achieve their optimum athletic performance. Electrolytes are molecules capable of conducting eletrical impulses and include sodium, potassium, calcium, magnesium, and chloride. Both muscle tissue and neurons are considered electric tissues of the body. Muscles and neurons are activated by electrolyte activity!

Muscle contraction is dependent upon the presence of calcium (Ca^{2+}), sodium (Na^+), and potassium (K^+). Without sufficient levels of these key electrolytes, muscle weakness or severe muscle contractions may occur.

Hyponatremia, a low concentration of sodium in the blood, has become more prevalent in ultra-endurance athletes. The Hawaii Ironman Triathlon routinely sees finishers with low blood sodium concentrations. Adequate sodium balance is necessary for transmitting nerve impulses and proper muscle function, and even a slight depletion of this concentration can cause problems. Ultra distance running events that take place in hot, humid conditions, and have athletes competing at high intensity have conditions prime for hyponatremia to develop.

During high intensity exercise, sodium is lost along with sweat. An athlete who only replaces the lost fluid with water may contribute to a decreased blood sodium concentration. Fluids with electrolytes are recommended for athletes during performance, especially during endurance events. It's also advisable to carry salt pills on a race. It's a good idea to take a salt pill (with water) at the start of specific muscle pain. For a good read on natural food sources of electrolytes See Hydration and Electrolytes - Impact on Athletic Performance by Paul Bennett, Jr. on 1Vigor.com

Hydration Needs of Runners, Hikers and Cyclists in Hot, Humid, Windy or Cold Weather. Once the body starts to become dehydrated, it can't function at its full capacity and as normal metabolism becomes impaired, your health and athletic performance is at risk. Dehydration risks increase during hot, humid, windy and cold weather.

Cold Weather Hydration. Surprisingly, dehydration is also a winter hazard. Sweat may not pour from your brow the way it does in summer, but depending on your level of exertion and the dryness of the air, significant moisture loss occurs. Also, fluid intake normally drops because people don't crave cold drinks during the winter.

The onset of dehydration often times is the cause of hypothermia. Hypothermia is very possible during endurance training and competitions (like Marathons and Ironman Triathlons) conducted in the cold. A person can become hypothermic if the rate of heat production during exercise is exceeded by the rate of heat loss. Dehydration and then Hypothermia causes a lower cellular metabolic rate which further decreases body temperature. During hypothermia blood volume decreases due to inadequate fluid intake reducing central nervous system and key organ functions.

Mountaineers are well aware drinking plenty of fluids during cold weather is essential to maintain core body temperatures to safely tackle the mountains in winter. Runners and cyclists should become equally aware of this need when training and racing in cold conditions.

Hot Weather Hydration. The debilitating effects of heat stress on the ability to perform prolonged strenuous exercise are well established. During exercise in a hot environment, a substantial rise in body core temperature is often linked with the onset of fatigue. Fluid replacement before and during prolonged exercise in the heat has been shown to be effective in reducing the elevation of body temperature and in extending endurance capacity.

Recent studies have show that ingestion of a cold drink before and during exercise in the heat reduced physiological strain (reduced heat accumulation) during exercise, leading to an improved endurance capacity. Exercise time was longer with the cold drink than with the warm drink, as the cold drink lowered heart rate, lowered skin and core temperature. Drinking cold drinks during exercise also reduced the need to sweat, resulting in a longer sweating capacity.

When exercising in hot weather, the combination of the external heat and the internal heat produced from the exercise, heat within the body can build causing Hyperthermia which is having a core body temperature that is too high. Maintaining good hydration can reduce the onset of Hyperthermia as good hydration enhances sweating which acts to cool core body temperatures.

Scientific data supports the position that caffeine reduces heat tolerance during exercise in a hot environment, via three physiological mechanisms. First, the diuretic effect of caffeine may exaggerate the declines that occur with plasma volume and stroke volume. Second, caffeine stimulates the sympathetic nervous system, and it may increase sweat rate. Third, caffeine increases resting metabolic rate in physically trained and sedentary individuals; this may increase heat storage and internal body temperature. These effects reduce heat tolerance (i.e., the exercise time to fatigue or exhaustion) by exacerbating dehydration and increasing body temperature. See How Caffeine Impacts Athletic Performance.

Humid Weather Hydration. In very humid weather, our sweat doesn't evaporate as very well and we tend to sweat more with less cooling effect thereby loosing needed fluids to maintain good performance. Fatigue will begin to increase when fluids are not replaced and under extreme lack of fluid replacement heat exhaustion or stroke can occur.

Windy Caused Dehydration. Windy conditions whether hot or cold can sap moisture from your body even when standing still. Extra hydration is necessary during windy conditions.

Acclimate. When training or racing in weather conditions very different from your training environment, it is recommendedl to arrive at the venue 4 days prior to the event, to enable the body to adjust to the different environment to reach a hydration balance consistent with this new environment.

4 NERVE FORCE

Breathing Rhythm For Optimum Health and Longevity. How we breath - our breathing rhythm - is one of the most important aspects of maintaining good health. Correct and proper breathing encourages optimum health and longevity. Fortunately, our breathing rhythm is something we have some control over. It's something we can change!

A healthy breathing rhythm is **deep, slow**, **quiet** and **regular**.

Optimum breathing rhythm can have the following benefits to good health:

- Calming.
- Regulates and balances our mental state.
- Sharpens focus. Practicing deep, slow, quiet and regular breathing can be a good exercise before athletic or other competition.
- Helps reduce our resting pulse rate. Improves blood circulation.
- Encourages metabolism efficiency.
- Fosters deep sleep.
- Harmonizes the function of our central nervous system.
- Enables more smooth functioning of our bodily organs.
- Allows men to enjoy greater stamina.

In some Eastern and Middle Eastern cultures and religion there is a belief that each of us are born with a certain number of breaths. There is some logic to this belief. Genetically, each of us are born with a certain energy destined to live and survive a certain length ot time. It's how we use and manage this energy - manage our metabolism - manage our lives, determines how long and how well we live. Proper breathing is a key tool to help manage our metabolism to live a better quality and longer life.

What is Healthy or Proper Breathing Technique? A healthy breathing rhythm is deep, slow, quiet and regular. Although breathing is involuntary, in that it occurs without our thinking about it, we also have some degree of control over our breathing. It is recommended we use our abdominal muscles and diaphram to inhale. By so doing, we are able to achieve the longest, slowest and deepest of breaths. We can also use our muscles to control our exhale to be long and slow.

Incidently, it is best to Inhale with our nose, as the primary functions of our nose is to (i) warm up air to body temperature through the moisture in our nose and (ii) filter and clean the air of particles.

Symptoms of Short or Shallow Breathing. When breathing in states of anger, breathing tends to be short, rapid, shallow and noisy. Short and shallow breathing can also cause less than adequate blood flow to the skin, panic attacks, panic disorders, anxiety, hypertension, frazzled nerves, cardiovascular stress, high blood pressure, stress, headaches, neck pain, fatigue, cold hands, and digestive and stomach disorders.

Breathing Properly a Natural Solution to help Solve Ailments. Proper breathing can play a role and may help solve many ailments without the need (or lessen the need) to take drugs and medications. Proper breathing can play a role and may also help you achieve normal functionality without the dependency on drugs and medications. It is worthy to note that many drugs may have toxicity implications and negative side effects.

Although learning proper breathing technique takes time, but over time, improving your breathing rhythm will work to make you more healthy.

When to Focus on Breathing. To improve your breathing rhythm, it is important to focus on slowing down your breathing rhythm regularly every day. A focus on your breathing and on breathing correctly can be very enjoyable. It can be done, for example, early in morning, when going to bed, when standing in a line, when in a meeting, when at a stop light, when waiting for a page to download on the internet, when pumping gas, when getting ready to take a power nap. You can add the productive task of focusing on your proper breathing during many tasks during the day.

Resting Pulse Rate an Indicator of Health, Fitness and Longevity. The purpose of this section is to (i) educate you on how your resting heart or pulse rate is a key measurement of your health, fitness level and lifespan, (ii) provide you with tips on how to lower your resting pulse rate (iii) teach you how to Measure your resting pulse rate, (iv) provide you with a Log to keep a record of your resting heart rate, and (v) help you be healthier and, if an athlete, improve athletic performance and reduce injury risk!

Why your Resting Heart Rate is Important to Track. As your resting pulse rate is a key vital sign and an important indicator of good health, it is important to be aware of and track your resting pulse rate for the following reasons:

- Longevity. At creation, each of us inherit a certain level of energy. How we manage that energy determines our lifespan. Those who have faster heart rates are using their heart beat allotment faster, therefore likely having a reduced lifespan.

- Faster Beat and Heart Attack Risk. A faster heart beat rate is a key indicator for the risk of heart attack.

Researchers have found that patients whose resting heart rate was above 70 beats per minute had significantly higher incidence of heart attacks.

- Strong Heart. A slower heart beat generally indicates a stronger heart that works less hard to pump blood throughout the body.

- Energy Levels. A slower heart rate generally indicates a longer, higher and more enduring energy levels

- Metabolic Efficiency. A slower required heart beat is a general indicator of an efficient metabolism.

- Athletic Endurance Fitness. A slower heart beat generally indicates aerobic fitness. Also, how quickly an athlete's heart beat recovers to lower beats per minute after vigorous exercise is an important indicator of aerobic fitness.

Managing your resting heart rate can be one of the most important things you can do to improve your lifespan and, for athletes, improve athletic performance.

What Impacts Resting Pulse Rate? The following impacts natural good sleep:

GOOD SLEEP. Have a routine of regularly getting good sleep. Regular disruptive or insufficient sleep is a significant contributor of a higher resting pulse rate. Full sleep enables the body to rest, repair and recovery.

REGULAR SUSTAINED AEROBIC EXERCISE. Regular sustained (at least an hour) of brisk aerobic exercise three times a week will help you maintain a lower resting pulse rate. Daily is better. Cycling, Hiking, walking, Swimming, Running are all good aerobic exercises to maintain a healthier resting pulse rate. Your aerobic exercise should be at a level to increase your heart rate. Researchers have found maintaining a Log encourages sticking with an exercise routine!

KEEP ARTERIES CLEAR THROUGH A NUTRITIOUS DIET. The clearer the arteries, the easier your blood with flow throughout your body. A healthy balanced diet consistency of natural organic unprocessed foods will help keep your arteries clear. It is also helpful to limit intake of excessively salty foods.

REDUCE and MANAGE EXCESS STRESS and ANXIETY. Stress can place extra burden on the heart and cardiovascular system. Living a Simple Lifestyle, learning techniques such as Yoga for Stress Management and appreciating the Vigor in Uncertainty are some effective things we can do to help keep our resting pulse rate in check.

STAY HYDRATED. Good hydration is key to keeping our blood at just the right viscosity to easily flow through our body, thus keeping our resting pulse rate in check. See Hydration Tips for Endurance Athletes for good information on hydration for everyone and under all weather conditions.

DON'T SMOKE. Smoking is hard on the heart and cardiovascular system.

MANAGE WEIGHT. Maintaining a good weight helps the body be efficient in the distribution of blood placing less stress on the heart.

LONG DEEP BREATHING. Long slow and deep breathing is a key way to reduce your resting heart rate. See Breathing Technique for Optimum Health

How and When to take a Resting Pulse Rate Measurement. Our resting heart rate is your heart rate when you are at rest, awake but lying down, and not having immediately exerted yourself. Resting pulse rate is measured by beats per minute (bpm). This measurement is best taken first thing in the morning before you get out of bed. Typical healthy resting heart rate in adults is 60–80 bpm. Note however that conditioned athletes often have resting heart rates below 60 bpm.

Tour de France cyclist Lance Armstrong has a resting HR around 32 bpm, and it is not unusual for people doing regular exercise to have resting pulse rates below 50 bpm.

The neck or wrist is a good place to find an artery with an easily noticable to the touch pulse to take your pulse rate with your finger!

It is very valuable to maintain a record of your resting pulse rate throughout your life as it can be an good hint and indicator of your overall health! 1Vigor.com has a cool free Log to track resting heart rate, as well as body fat %, hours of sleep, weight and aerobic activities such as walking, hiking, running, swimming, cycling and kayaking. The Log can also track yoga, pushups, situps, pullups and weight lifting.

It is a good idea to measure and record your resting pulse rate at least once a week!

Athletes Manage Resting Pulse Rate for Improve Performance. Managing your Resting Heart Rate is an imporant training tool for athletes for the following reasons:

- Take Resting Pulse Rate in the morning of a long workout day. Adjust your workout intensity if your resting pulse rate is too high that morning. A higher than average resting pulse rate may indicate a period of inadequate rest.
- Monitor your Resting Pulse Rate during your Tapering Period prior to your Race. Adjust your tapering intensity in part based upon your resting pulse rate. Pre race excitement aside, it is best race morning to have your resting pulse rate within your usual low range. A higher resting pulse rate race morning may make for a long day.
- Regularly Monitor your Resting Pulse Rate as a Way to Prevent Overtraining. Overtraining can lower your immune system, cause you to become ill and can

increase your risk of injury. . . . all of which may cut into your training time. Your resting pulse rate is an excellent easy and quick indicator to prevent overtraining. It may also signal the need for more rest.

Natural Sleep Rejuvenates the Mind and Body. When we sleep well naturally (without drugs or pills), we wake up feeling refreshed and alert for our daily activities. Sleep affects how we look, feel and perform on a daily basis. Sleep directly impacts our overall quality of life. An average of regularly scheduled 8 hours of deep sleep each day is essential to reaping the full benefits of deep sleep. Good quantity and quality of sleep leaves our bodies and minds rejuvenated for the next day. Full sleep enables needed muscle repair, memory consolidation and the release of hormones regulating growth and appetite. Full sleep enables us to be prepared to concentrate, make decisions, and be engaged fully in all our activities.

Ten Ways Sleep Rejuvenates the Body:

- Blood pressure drops, breathing slows and muscles relax which gives the nervous system an opportunity to rest
- The Growth Hormone and other hormones are released into the blood stream to promote growth and development
- Blood supply to the muscles increases
- Tissue growth and repair occurs including muscle growth and repair
- Energy is restored
- The Immune System is strengthened
- Energy is restored
- Rapid Eye Movement sleep occurs (REM sleep), which accounts for 25% of our sleep, providing energy to the brain and the body.
- Carbohydrates fuel the brain with Brain Nutrition

13 Tips to Good Sleep Naturally.   Good sleep is earned. Here are 13 Tips to Good Sleep Naturally:

- Long and deep breathing sets the stage for the body to wind down to enable falling asleep quickly
- Living a life of Integrity, self respect and respect of others enables sleep with a clear conscience
- Living a Simple Life, but a rich life
- Vigorous Exercise for at least an hour a day insures the body will be tired at night
- A day of Hard Work, Stimulation and Challenge
- Setting and accomplishing daily and long term Goals, creates a sense of Peace and Satisfaction when night arrives
- Avoiding negative thoughts and worries
- Sleeping with the Window Open
- Sleeping in a cool room is helpful because body temperature drops during sleep. Sleeping too warmly increases the pulse rate which then makes it more difficult for the body to relax enough to sleep soundly
- A cup of Milk helps the body relax and its carbohydrates fuel the brain and provide Brain Nutrition
- Eat healthy foods
- Eat very little within two hours of bedtime
- Sleep in Darkness. Sleeping in complete darkness is important to getting a good night's sleep because darkness increases the production of Melatonin. Melatonin is a hormone produced by the pineal gland in the brain and controls the body's sleeping cycle. Melatonin is believed to cause us to fall asleep faster and sleep better.

Beat Depression Natually.   Do Antidepressants Cure Depression? Although the human experience can be filled with much wonder, deep learning and insight, great achievement, intense love, joy and happiness, and a sense of belonging, the human condition is also filled with loneliness, hardship, setback, failure, disappointment, sadness, loss, challenge, adversity and stress. Change, challenge, adversity and stress is a core foundation of the natural universe and is experienced by all living things. This stress in many respects is and should be considered positive. Stress and adversity provide challenge, sharpen skills, build strength and the opportunities to improve.

Most of us experience various degrees of depression at different points in our lives. Unfortunately, in recent years, too many in our medical and therapist communities have embraced offering prescription mood altering drugs, anti-depressants, tranquillizers and sleeping pills to their patients, instead of first and primarily recommending natural solutions to combat depression, as if these pills are a solution or cure to the underlying conditions causing depression. "Significant increases in antidepressant use were evident across all sociodemographic groups . . . ." Dr. Mark Olfson of Columbia University in New York and Steven Marcus of the University of Pennsylvania in Philadelphia wrote in the Archives of General Psychiatry. "Not only are more U.S. residents being treated with antidepressants, but also those who are being treated are receiving more antidepressant prescriptions," they added. About 6 percent of people were prescribed an antidepressant in 1996 -- 13 million people. This rose to more than 10 percent or 27 million people by 2005, these researchers found.

In the United States, a pill dependent culture is being created with the encouragement by many school officials, and many in the drug, medical and therapist communities to provide mood altering and anti-depressant drugs to boys and young men with high energy levels. Might these boys and young men be better served by being encouraged to funnel that energy into playing sports, play chess or study the sciences!

Studies have indicated that antidepressants do not cure depression or provide a remedy for the underlying conditions that cause depression, except in the most severe cases. Very recent research of efficacy trials submitted to the US Food and Drug Administration (FDA) suggests that antidepressants are only "marginally efficacious" compared with placebo and "document profound publication bias that inflates their apparent efficacy." Very recent studies have also found that Antidepressant medications offer significant benefit in the treatment of the severest depressive symptoms, but may have little or no therapeutic benefit in patients with mild to moderate depression — a population which accounts for most cases. A purpose of this page is not to be critical of those taking antidepressants and antipsychotic medications, but to provide insight into natural alternatives to those that don't need them and to perhaps lessen the need/dosage for those that do.

Antidepressant's Harmful Side Effects. Most of these antidepressant, tranqualizers and mood altering pills:

1. DO NOT address the underlying reasons for the depression.

2. DUMB DOWN and depress the nervous system in many instances causing the patients senses to be less aware of reality. (How effective can one be in dealing with reality when dumbed down to it?)

3. HAVE SERIOUS SIDE EFFECTS including nausea, increased weight gain (due to disruption to their natural Metabolism), loss of sexual drive, insomnia, dry mouth, fatigue, agitation and anxiety.

4. CAN CREATE DEPENDENCY and DO NOT help people be real and deal with life's challenges and stress. I'm of the opinion, the above drugs should only be used as a very last resort to treat depression, anxiety, or insomnia which is severe and chronic, i.e. when the person's day to day functioning is badly affected and where the problem is not responsive to any other forms of treatment. Many times, however, prescription drugs are

the first line of treatment and this often becomes an obstacle in the road to health, wellbeing and balance. When one becomes depressed the natural ways to fight depression should be considered.

14 Tips to Beat Depression Naturally. Here are a few good tips to help naturally fight depression:

1. Set Short and Long Term Goals. Define your purposes in life. Then set short and long term goals and a plan to accomplish these purposes.

2, Socialize and Build Meaningful Relationships When you are depressed, you usually isolate yourself and avoid company. Mixing with people is not always what you feel like doing, but loneliness is one of the major causes of depression. Get out there and join the world! You may hate it at first, but do it anyway! It will ultimately help to uplift your spirits and you will not feel so alone. If you don't have a social circle, join one! Volunteer organizations, mothers' groups, churches, chess or sports clubs, hobbies and crafts are all good ideas. Take on a responsbility involving Leadership. Be creative! Try out different alternatives until you find something that you like. Don't give up!

3. Loneliness is a Natural State, but extended Loneliness causes Depression There is a basic human need to connect and when that need is not met we can become lonely. Each of us are alone at a certain level. Through all phases of life we will experience loneliness. Lonliness is part of the human condition. Being lonely isn't bad for you, but staying lonely is. Loneliness has repercussions on health and wellbeing and can cause sleep dysfunction and higher blood pressure. Loneliness comes down to quality not quantity of friendships. It's not the number of relationships that impacts loneliness, but the quality of those relationships that determine whether you feel socially isolated. In a quality way . . . . . Connect!

4. Have a Nutritious Diet. Eat healthy. Eat natural foods pack with nutrients captured from sun's energy like Vegetables and Fruits and Whole Grains. Some foods help to fight depression and anxiety. A carbohydrate rich diet helps the body produce serotonin - the 'feelgood' chemical. Special serotonin foods are oats, pasta, whole wheat, bananas and other carbohydrate rich foods. A cup of Milk before bedtime makes for a good night sleep and provides Brain Nutrition.

Make sure you are having a full supplement of Vitamin D, Vitamin B, magnesium, zinc and iron - a deficiency in any of these can lead to depression and anxiety-type symptoms and insomnia. Good hydration helps keep the body and the mind in balance.

Vitamine D Sources: The Sun, cod liver oil, salmon, mackerel, tuna, sardines, milk, eggs, liver, and cheese. See also Vitamin D Synthesis from the Sun and Food Sources.

Vitamin B12 Sources: Mollusks, clams, liver, beef, yogurt, milk, eggs, chicken. Vitamin B6 Sources: Potato, banana, garbanzo beans, chicken, oatmeal, beef spinach, salmon, wheat bran, peanut butter. Niacin Sources: Chicken, turkey, beef, salmon, whole wheat bread, yeast, pasta, peanuts, lentils, and lima beans. Folate Sources: Beef, liver, peas, pasta, spinach, asparagus, rice, broccoli, egg noodles, avocado, peanuts, wheat germ, tomato juice, orange juice, whole wheat bread, eggs, cantaloupe, papaya, and banana.

Iron Sources: Chicken livers, oysters, beef, Turkey, chicken, halibut, tuna, shrimp, pasta, oatmeal, soybeans, lentils, beans, molasses, spinach, peas, grits, raisins, whole wheat bread. Magnesium Sources: Halibut, almonds, cashews, spinach, oatmeal, potato, peanuts, peas, yogurt, rice, lentils, avocado, beans, banana, milk, whole wheat bread, and raisins.

A traditional or whole diet characterized by vegetables, fruit, whole grains, and high-quality meat and fish may help prevent mental illness — specifically, depression and anxiety. Conversely, a Western diet high in refined or processed foods and saturated fats may increase the risk of depression, new research suggests.

5. Help Others. Step back, focus away from your concerns and needs for a moment and look around. Everyone has stress, challenges and is faced with adversity. Reach out to help others in need. There is an emotional aspect to gratitude which creates a desire to give to others. Giving to others connects you to others and your community.

6. Exercise and Get Outdoors
Regular sustained (at least an hour) of brisk aerobic exercise three times a week will help you realize Aerobic Health Benefits. Daily is better if you are trying to beat depression. Cycling, Hiking, walking, Swimming, Running, dance, aerobics, etc. This aerobic exercise should be at a level to increase your heart rate. Exercise enhances and increases blood flow to each cell and to the vital organs bringing more oxygen and more nutrients to both and improving the cell performance and organ function. Exercise strengthens metabolism, extends our life's 'battery' and builds cell, organ and metabolic efficiency. Learning a sport builds confidence. Exercise makes us happy. Keeping a Log encourages an Exercise Routine! Being Outdoors and exploring nature is also a great way to relax, feel good, break from your routine, get Vitamin D and earn a good night sleep. Being in a hike in nature may be one of the best ways to brighten the spirit. Vitamin D deficiency is considered to be a contributing factor causing depression.

7. Simplify Your Life But Have Adventure, Challenge and Variety If your depression is caused in part by having a complex life that causes worry, it's a good ideal to simplify your life. Extreme worry destroys health, damages the immune system and weakens the cardiovascular and nervous system. A simple life,

and that does not mean a dull or boring life, is a life of lower worries and better worry management. Take on a challenge. Challenge helps focus the mind. Add adventure to your routine.

Routines get boring. I've found that one of the most ultimately relaxing experiences I've had is rock climbing. The intense but complete focus on the simple but important task of optimum hand and foot placement during times of some risk and danger unclutters the mind of all worry and distraction. I've experience real peace and clarity after rock climbing. This is not a recommendation for everyone to rock climb, as rock climbing is not meant for everyone. However, it is a good example of how taking on a challenge that requires some intense focus (it could be playing chess) has a way of clearing the mind of static.

8. Good Sleep Patterns. When we sleep well naturally (without drugs or pills), we wake up feeling refreshed and alert for our daily activities. Sleep affects how we look, feel and perform on a daily basis. Sleep directly impacts our overall quality of life. An average of regularly scheduled 8 hours of deep sleep each day is essential to reaping the full benefits of deep sleep. Good quantity and quality of sleep leaves our bodies and minds rejuvenated for the next day. Full sleep enables needed muscle repair, memory consolidation and the release of hormones regulating growth and appetite. Full sleep enables us to be prepared to concentrate, make decisions, and be engaged fully in all our activities. Lack of regular good sleep can cause depression and feelings of being overwhelmed.

9. Be Thankful for What You Have. All of us have things we can be thankful of. Taking stock of your strengths, abilities, and positive situation offers a foundation upon which you can think positively about yourself. From this positive foundation you can build upon a sense of appreciation and gratitude. With a sense of gratitude and thankfulness you can place in proper perspective feelings of dysfunction, anger, regret, loss, imbalance, misfortune and other negative emotions and thoughts. Adopting a sense of gratitude and thankfulness can be an excellent coping mechanism

during stressful conditions. There is a power that comes from thankfulness and positive thinking.

10. Get Over it! You are going to run into roadblocks and carry many negative thoughts. You know what these negative thoughts are. We all experience negative thoughts. But, Knock it off! Got over it and move on! Be accountable for yourself. Pull your own strings.

11. Develop Relaxation skills. Relaxation techniques and meditation are easy to learn and are so effective in relieving stress, anxiety, and depression. Meditation is a form of mental discipline that encompasses a wide range of spiritual and/or psychophysical practices, each emphasizing different goals. Developing Meditation skills can be a good tool to fighting depression as mediation can help develop greater focus, creativity, better self-awareness, mental clarity and can improve brain chemistry. Certain breathing rhythm and techniques create relaxation. See Breathing Technique for Optimum Health

12. Smile and Laugh. Smile! Laugh! Laugh at yourself.

13. For Men: Keep Testosterone Levels Up! There is considerable evidence of an association with depressive symptoms and low testosterone levels in men. See Amiaz, Kanayama, Pope, Seidman "Testosterone Supplementation for Depressed Men: Current Research and Suggested Treatment Guidelines" Experimental and Clinical Psychopharmacology 2007, Vol. 15, No. 6, pages 529-538. See How to Increase Testosterone Naturally

14. Quit Smoking! Mental illness and depression are associated with both higher rates of smoking and higher levels of smoking among smokers. Further, a significant proportion of smokers have mental illness or depression.

How I Quit Smoking Cigarettes. When I was 19, I smoked over a pack of cigarettes each day and found myself tired walking up a flight of stairs. Tired at age 19! One night driving along the Long Island Expressway, the following lyrics from "I am the Walrus", by the Beatles, caught my attention: "Expert textpert choking smokers, Don't you think the joker laughs at? See how they smile like pigs in a sty, see how they snied. I'm crying." In other words, tobacco companies were making profits from my cigarette habit which was taking life from me slowly. Today, the cigarette profiteers are government who are happy to collect significant tax revenues from cigarette sales while the smoking is killing us slowly. I realized, while driving home, John, Paul, George and Ringo were right. I ripped in half my pack of cigarettes and have not had a cigarette since. It was hard quiting! But, I substituted something I did not like that was healthy in its stead . . . yogurt. Now I can eat 8 yogurts (plain) a day.

Harmful Impact of Smoking. Nicotine, the primary psychoactive chemical in cigarettes, has been shown to be addictive. 1. Statistically each cigarette smoked shortens the user's lifespan by 11 minutes. 2. About half of cigarette smokers die of tobacco-related disease and lose on average 14 years of life. 3. Cigarette smoking causes depression. 4. In men, cigarette smoking lowers testosterone and causes the genitals to shrink! 5.Cigarette use by pregnant women has also been shown to cause mental and physical birth defects. 6. Causes sleep loss.

Tips to Quit Smoking Naturally. Here are some good tips to help you quit smoking cigarettes naturally:

1.Substitute Something Healthy instead to eat or do. Find a food that is healthy, natural and low calorie.

2. Get Angry that government and tobacco companies profit slowly taking life from you! REFUSE TO BE A VICTIM.

3. Engage in an Aerobic Sport like Cycling, Hiking, walking, Swimming, Running, or dance or sign up for an aerobics class.

4. (having fun) Listen to/watch video of I am the Walrus.

5. Find a Buddy that can help you when the urge arises to smoke. Build a support system.

6. Others need you. Realize that others need you to be at your best.

7. Value your life. We are not meant to live a life of being sick, run down and under the weather often. Good health will improve the quality of your life and your giving to others.

8. Develop an aversion to the smell and taste of tobacco and smoke. Recognize how this smell permeates your skin, hair, clothing and furniture and develop an aversion and dislike for the smell.

9. Occupy your hands and mouth with items other than cigarettes like carrot sticks.

10. Drink plenty of fluids to help your body begin to flush out nicotine from its system.

11. Professional, Medical Help and Aids. Where the addiction is very strong, there is medical and professional help, and over the counter and prescription aids to help you quit smoking.

5 BRAIN POWER

Brain Nutrition. The brain is a complex organ that has unique nutrient needs. Good nutrition for the brain calls for a diet low in saturated fats and sugars, and high in foods rich in vitamin B. The brain needs glucose, proteins, fatty acids, vitamins, minerals and other essential nutrients to run at peak performance. Glucose for is the brain's fuel, so an adequate intake of carbohydrates is essential for optimall brain function. Glucose is obtained by eating carbohydrates and other foods that can be converted to glucose.

To maximize brain performance it is important to eat quality carbohydrates from whole grains, fruits and vegetables and dairy products. Empty carbohydrates consumed from refined sugar products are not a good source of brain fuel. Milk, Eggs, liver, meats, fish and legumes are an essential source of brain fuel. To function well, your brain needs a good supply of essential fatty acids known as omega-3.

The brain needs glucose, proteins, fatty acids, vitamins, minerals and other essential nutrients to run at peak performance. Since the body cannot produce these fatty acids, you need to get them from food. These fatty acids are found in fish oils, nuts, and seeds. Consume more eggs. Eggs are an excellent source of dietary choline. Choline a necessary component of two fat-like molecules in the brain, phosphatidylcholine and sphingomyelin. They help maintain brain health.

Top 10 Brain Foods Here is a list of the top ten brain foods that are either rich in the Omega-3 fatty acid, protein and vitamin B's and/or quality carbohydrates.

Top 10 Brain Foods:
1. Salmon
2. Eggs
3. Peanut Butter
4. Whole Grains
5. Oats/Oatmeal
6. Berries
7. Beans
8. Colorful Veggies
9. Milk and Yogurt
10. Lean Beef and Chicken

Learning and Intelligence. What is Intelligence? Intelligence is a biopsychological process that is a product of genetic heritage and psychological properties ranging from personality dispositions to cognitive powers. Intelligence is a combination of the ability to: (i) Learn. This includes all kinds of informal and formal learning via any combination of experience, education, and training. (ii) Pose problems. This includes recognizing problem situations and transforming them into more clearly defined problems. (iii) Solve problems. This includes solving problems, accomplishing tasks creating, fashioning products, and doing complex projects. The good news is that the definition of intelligence implies the ability to improve. It says that each of us can become more intelligent. We can become more intelligent through desire and determination, study and practice, through access to appropriate tools, and through learning to make effective use of these tools.

The Different Types of Intelligence. It is recognized that we all have a multiple of intelligences, with no two intelligences being the same, as we each have a unique degree of the differing intelligences. Some recognized intelligences are:

- Musical Intelligence which is the ability to learn, perform, and compose music.

- Bodily-Kinesthetic Intelligence which is the ability to use one's physical body well.

- Logical-Mathematical Intelligence which is the ability to learn higher mathematics. The ability to handle complex logical arguments.

- Linguistic Intelligence which is the ability to communicate well, perhaps both orally and in writing, perhaps in several languages.

- Spatial Intelligence which is the ability to know where you are relative to fixed locations. The ability to accomplish tasks requiring three-dimensional visualization and placement of your hands or other parts of your body.

- Interpersonal Intelligence which is the core capacity to notice distinctions in others, particularly moods, temperament, motivations and intentions. The ability to discern the intentions and desires of others even when hidden. Intrapersonal Intelligence is the knowledge of the internal aspects of oneself. The ability to sense other's feelings and be in tune with others. The ability to access to ones own feeling and life, ones range of emotions, and the capacity to make discrimination among the range of emotions as a means to guide and understand ones behavior. A person with good intrapersonal intelligence has an effective model of himself consistent with a description constructed by careful observers. The self-awareness ability to know your own body and mind.

- Naturalistic Intelligence which is the ability to understand different species, recognize patterns in nature, classify natural objects.

- Neural Intelligence which is the ability to have insight into one's efficiency and precision of one's neurological system.
- Experiential intelligence which refers to one's accumulated knowledge and experience in different areas. It can be thought of as the accumulation of all of one's expertises.
- Reflective Intelligence. This refers to one's broad-based strategies for attacking problems, for learning, and for approaching intellectually challenging tasks. It includes attitudes that support persistence, systemization, and imagination. It includes self-monitoring and self-management.
- Reflexive intelligence can be thought of as a control system that helps to make effective use of neural intelligence and experiential intelligence. A person can learn strategies that help to make more effective use of neural intelligence and experiential intelligence. The habits of mind included under reflexive intelligence can be learned and improved.
- Existential Intelligence which is the ability to discern and understand the big questions of life and the most fundamental questions of existence.

Creativity Skills for a Vigorous Lifestyle. Creativity makes for a more vigorous lifestyle, enhances longevity and help builds strong brain power. Creativity increases arousal and heightens the senses and awareness. Creativity engages passion, encourages purpose, sharpens goals and enacts ideas into productive valuable concrete results. Carpe Diem was common greeting in Ancient Rome. This Latin term means "Seize the Day" and has been embraced by modern culture to remind us to live each moment of the day joyously, alive, aware and productively.

What is Creativity? Creative means original and of high quality. Creativity is producing something of value. Creativity is the driving force that turns dreams into reality. Creativity happens when we are in a curious, receptive, open and humble state of mind. Creativity happens when boundaries are removed, or at least extended, and we become enabled to tap into something bigger than ourselves. Creativity is making oneself less separate, tuning into currents of change and then seizing the opportunity to become the messenger that creates value to others. Creativity plays with the (seemingly) impossible and is the spice of life.

Creativity is a skill of the Brain which has three primary steps. 1. Imagination.

1. The first step in Creativity is to imagine. This initial step is about letting your imagination go wild and dreaming up as many ideas. This step is about freeing your brain to dream up lots of ideas. Ideas need to be first caught and then refined.

2. Critique. The second step in Creativity is to critique the ideas imagined in the first step. Brainstorming and collecting the input from a diverse group of people is an excellent way to critique ideas. Brainstorming gathers a mix of broader ideas and different perspectives which will stimulate idea generation and improve the idea. A good brainstorming environment occurs where negative criticism is suspended and there exists a nonjudgmental attitude. Each new person added to the brainstorming process creates exponential new possibilities and relationships.

3. Enactment. The third step is enactment of the idea. Creativity is more than just using your imagination. After critical thinking and improvement of the idea, a skill in itself, hard work, discipline and fortitude are needed to enact the idea into a valuable product or creation. This stage of enactment combines real life skills to turn your ideas into success.

There is a concept called Creative Discontent which holds that Creativity is the natural evolution of things driven by a sense that things can always be or be done better. Creativity is driven by competition and the desire to improve.

Innovation and Physiology. Physiology has an important affect on innovation and imagination potential. It can have a very positive or very negative impact on imagination. Fatigue and stress stunt imagination. Good sleep makes for an alert brain which is imagination's best friend.

Negative stress like worry lower's your level of concentration and stifles your imagination. It can also lower your ability to critique ideas and plan them. Positive stress like deadlines and the excitement of new ventures and creations heighten the senses and improve imagination. Alcohol and drugs are depressants which slows your body's cognitive and motor functions and blocks inhibition. Good nutrition can play an important role in improving creativity.

Exercise and Creativity. Creativity is informally considered to play a key role in the attractiveness and competitiveness of individuals and organizations. Exercise enhances cognitive functioning. Research on this aspect of cognitive functioning has often found a positive relationship between physical exercise and creativity. Exercise has been shown to have positive effects on physiological arousal and attention narrowing, as well as creativity. Research has shown that aerobic exercise for an hour or two has an immediate and enduring effect of significantly increasing creativity potential. Individuals realize greater gains from aerobic exercise, but their families, employers, communities and organizations may potentially benefit as well. However, it is good to note that excessive exercise can cause fatigue which can have the debilitating effect of depressing arousal and creativity.

Creativity Traits. Creativity traits includes fluency, flexibility, originality, elaboration, curiosity, imagination, complexity, risk taking, discipline, fortitude and attention to purpose.

Heightened Senses and Expanded Awareness Improve Performance, Arousal and Life Quality. Our brain power is enhanced when we become more aware of the things around us. Increasing our awareness and arousal is accomplished by increasing our sensitivity to our senses. Heightened sense sensitivity occurs with increased concentration on the senses while at the same time clearing the mind of distractions to enable a more sharpened focus. Meditation or Yoga provides a good vehicle to sharpen awareness of the senses.

Heightened Senses, Metabolism and Longevity. Heightened sense awareness is important to the quality of our life and important to achieving longevity and a longer lifespan for a few reasons. First, increased sense awareness enables a more efficient Metabolism. Second, increased sense awareness requires us to become more in tune and connected with our metabolism. Third, increased sense awareness increases the sensitivity to pulse rate and benefits to correct deep breathing. Fourth, increased sense awareness enables us to perform life responsibilities more richly resulting in an increased sense of competency and corresponding increase in confidence. Fifth, increased sense awareness regarding time enables one to better manage our metabolism and maintain a high metabolism all for the purpose of extending our lifespan.

The Five Basic and Other Senses. Here are our five basic senses, the energy form detected, and their related body parts are and other senses:

- Sight - Light energy detected by the eyes.
- Hearing - Sound energy detected by the ears.
- Smell - Chemical energy and shape of molecules detected by the nose.
- Taste - Chemical energy detected by the tongue.

- Touch - Pressure energy detected by the skin. Additional Senses
- Sixth Sense - Psychic energy detected by the brain.
- Time – '4th Dimension' energy detected by the brain
- Temperature - Heat energy detected by skin but with different nerve endings than for the sense of touch.
- Balance - Gravity energy detected by inner ear.
- Electrical Fields – Electric energy detected by the brain and other senses.
- Magnetic Fields – Earth's magnetic energy detected by the brain.

The Sense of Time. There are different measures of time, including the apparent motion of the sun across the sky, the phases of the moon, the swing of a pendulum, and the beat of our heart. Currently, the international unit of time, the second, is defined in terms of radiation emitted by caesium atoms. Our sense of time is also impacted by the Circadian clock (Our 24 hour clock set by the location of the sun). This 'clock' has various psychophysiological factors that influences our perception of time. Our working memory loads, time of day, body temperature, and mood are considered important modifiers of our perception of time. The perception of time is also impacted by hormones such as adrenaline. In stressful situations where adrenaline is increased into the bloodstream, time seems to go into slow motion and there exists an ability to vividly recall events for a long time after. Increased adrenaline increases awareness.

How the Experience of Slow Motion Impacts Awareness. It seems that in certain important or dangerous situations, perception of time goes into slow motion, such that a person is aware of everything happening at a different rate of time than what is normal. People have experienced this when engaged in special occasions, giving a speech, being involved in a car accident, or falling from a tree or similar event time seems to slow or stand still. Experiencing the world more frequently in relative slow motion is a valuable skill to improve our awareness as it requires and builds a greater focus and more sharp senses. People that live in the moment or are in the 'zone' usually have sharpened their awareness skills.

Do Humans have Electrical Fields? All living organisms, including humans, are thought to have electrical fields. This electrical field is sometimes referred to as 'Aura''. Humans have an aura which is a result of all our metabolic processes including those that result in electrical impulses such as muscle contraction, heart beat and brain signals. The electrical signals that come from your muscles, heart, brain and other parts of your body create an electrical field. There is also an energy that flows from emotions which are psychophysiological. There is thought regarding ones electrical signals that when your senses are heightened and when your mind and heart are in harmony, your electrical signals are in synch and strong. This harmony results in an apparent better health and a stronger personal aura, presence and attractiveness.

Clear Thinking Skills. Clear Thinking plays an important role in our Lifestyle and Longevity. The higher our thought clarity the better will be our ability to perceive, solve problems, create and be self-aware. In turn, Clear Thinking skills translate into making smarter decisions regarding our life's purpose, personal achievements, and interpersonal relationships. Clear Thinking improves the contributions we make to our play, work, employment, and contributions to society. Clear Thinking improves our lifestyle. Clear Thinking improves Longevity because it enables a more efficient Metabolism, a metabolism focused on the long term.

What is Clear Thinking? Clear Thinking is the ability to think critically and rationally with the ability to engage in independent and reflective thought. Clear Thinking is not just a matter of accumulating information. A person with a good memory is not necessarily a good clear thinker. A clear thinker is able to deduce consequences from what is known, and knows how to make use of information to solve problems. Clear Thinking can help us acquire knowledge and make better life decisions.

Clear Thinking skills includes the ability to:

- understand the logical connections between ideas
- identify, construct and evaluate arguments
- detect inconsistencies and common mistakes in reasoning
- solve problems systematically by correctly using information
- identify the relevance and importance of ideas
- perceive accurately
- hypothesize
- be emotionally aware
- reflect on the justification of one's own beliefs and values
- think quickly

According to Dr. Peter A. Facione, Critical Thinking: What It Is and Why It Counts, "The ideal critical thinker is habitually inquisitive, well-informed, trustful of reason, open-minded, flexible, fair minded in evaluation, honest in facing personal biases, prudent in making judgments, willing to reconsider, clear about issues, orderly in complex matters, diligent in seeking relevant information, reasonable in the selection of criteria, focused in inquiry, and persistent in seeking results which are as precise as the subject and the circumstances of inquiry permit".

What is the Clear Thinking State of Mind? Once clear thinking skills are improved and mastered it is then important to exercise those skills in the best possible state of mind for optimum clear thinking. The optimum state of mind for clear thinking is similar to the Ideal Performance State under which athletes are able to achieve at peak performance.

The Ideal Performance State is:

* Personally challenged
* Energized with positive emotions
* Ready for fun and enjoyment
* Focused and alert
* On automatic instinct
* Relaxed and calm
* Maintaining confidence

What are Valuable Intellectual Traits? Richard Paul and Linda Elder, Foundation of Critical Thinking have identified the following intellectual traits that provide a framework to discipline and improve mental functioning:

-Intellectual Humility
-Intellectual Courage
-Intellectual Empathy
-Intellectual Integrity
-Intellectual Perseverance
-Faith In Reason
-Fair-mindedness

Clear Thinking and Physiology. The brain utilizes a significant portion of our total energy to perform. While resting and quietly awake, the brain consumes about 20% of our metabolism even though the brain represents only 2% of the total body weight. During active periods, the brain can consume up to 30% of caloric intake. Since the brain consumes such a large percentage of the body's energy, it is physiologically important to have a clear mind so that brain energy is not wasted. Clear Thinking is efficient thinking and from a physiologic standpoint focus energy more productively. Clear Thinking that does not waste brain energy also helps in the overall objective of maintaining an efficient metabolism. Having an efficient metabolism is an important element of achieving longevity.

Self-Actualization Skills to Improve Lifestyle and Athletic Performance. Self-Actualization is a key component in enhancing vigor, improving brain power, building stronger relationships, becoming a better athlete and achieving longevity. Self Actualization is a continual process of growth and a source of pride and happiness. A richer lifestyle and longer healthier life can be an achievement of Self-Actualization.

What is Self-Actualization? Self-actualization is a level of development where personal growth becomes an psychological needs. Self-Actualization is an enduring driving force with us. It's been said that all examples of people who achieve greatness or do great things share an inner inspiration to express their soul potential.

Self-Actualization has been identified as the highest need in Abraham Maslow's Hierarchy of Needs and includes the Self-Actualization of benefitting others:

PHYSIOLOGICAL - Basic living needs, such as food, water, oxygen and sex.
SAFETY - Once physiological needs are satisfied, you need to have a home and other forms of security.
BELONGING - So far you have taken care of yourself. Once you do this, you look to make friends, find someone to love and in general feel part of a community.
SELF-ESTEEM - You need self-confidence, to be appreciated for what you are and be treated with dignity.
SELF-ACTUALIZATION. This is the highest level. Once your basic needs are supplied, you seek ways to reach your highest potential.

Self-Actualization is the essence of human nature. As Dr. Maslow found, "practically every human being, and certainly in almost every newborn baby, that there is an active will toward health, an impulse towards growth, or towards actualization".

How is Self-Actualization Realized? After the basic human needs, such as food, shelter, clothing, health, and employment needs are met, our needs of friendship, family, and sexual intimacy. Humans also need to feel a sense of belonging and acceptance from social groups, such as clubs, work, religious groups, professional organizations, sports teams, family, intimate partners, mentors, close colleagues, and confidants. After these physiological, safety, belonging, social and esteem needs are meet, we by nature seek to grow through Self-Actualization.

What are the Barriers to Self-Actualization? The following can be barriers to Self-Actualization:

- Ignorance. Self-mastery is essentially impossible if one is not willing to devote time to understanding the nature of the mind.
- Negative Habit Formation. Being stuck in a set behaviors and patterns of thought that do not support our pursuit of worldly success or self-mastery.
- Destructive Personality Traits. Low self esteem trains such as self-destruction, self-indulgence and self-pity.
- Ego Defense Mechanisms. Our Ego is subject to a number of self-deceptions preventing self-mastery that manifest as a stressful emotional state such as fear, guilt, embarrassment, anger, or frustration.
- Negative Self-Talk. Thoughts have a great impact on the emotions, feelings or states of mind that is operate at any given moment of time.
- Arrested Development. Ego growth has stopped prematurely.

- Failure to Master Negative Emotions and States of Mind.
- Poor Attention Management and Self-Awareness. One must properly focus attention to process any type of information.

Characterizations of Self-Actualizing People. Here are some characteristics of Self-Acutalizing people:

- Realistically oriented and not threatened by the unknown.
- Superior ability to reason and to see the truth.
- Perceive and understand human nature.
- Self accept and acceptance of other people, circumstances and the natural world. for what they are.
- Ability to learn from anyone and are friendly with anyone.
- Emotionally intelligent and feel no need for crippling guilt or shame.
- Serene. Self starters who are responsible for themselves and own their behavior.
- Work becomes play
- Retain dignity amid confusion and personal misfortune.
- Spontaneous and have no unnecessary inhibitions.
- The self-actualized person can be alone and not be lonely.
- Honest and seek justice for all.
- Autonomous and independent.
- Moment to moment living for them is exciting and often exhilarating as they live their life to the full.
- Seek wholeness.
- Retain childlike qualities.
- Have a far-seeing wisdom.
- Intimate relationships tend to be profound, sincere and long-lasting.

- Maintain an inborn uniqueness.
- Motivated to continual growth.
- Enthusiastic about life.

The good news is that despite our genetic makeup, environment and experiences, we can all improve upon our ability to Self-Actualize and reach our potential!

6 MEN'S UNIQUE HEALTH ISSUES

How to Raise Testosterone Levels and Production Naturally. The purpose of this section is to (i) educate you on the role testosterone plays in men's health and (ii) provide information to help you naturally keep your testosterone levels up so you will be stronger and live longer, and (iii) help you be a better athlete!!

What is Testosterone? Testosterone is the hormone that gives men their male characteristics. Testosterone give men their a deep voice, higher muscle mass, facial and torso hair, and aggressive behaviour. Testosterone also is the hormone that controls sexual function in men. Testosterone is know for its ability to increase libido. Testosterone also plays a key role in keeping men's bones dense and strong and in building muscle mass.

When do Testosterone Levels Begin to Decrease? Testosterone levels are at the highest during puberty and adolescence when boys physically change to young men. However, testosterone levels begin declining after the age of 30. This decline leads to many changes in your body. The normal level of testosterone in your bloodstream is between 350 and 1,000 nanograms per deciliter (ng/dl).Testosterone begins declining after the age of 30 and research indicates that in an average men generally lose 1% of testosterone a year.

This decline is testosterone levels is gradual but on average by the time you reach 40 you have already lost 10% of this hormone and you can feel the effects more sharply. Testosterone levels in American men have been declining steadily over the past two decades, according to a 2006 study in the Journal of Clinical Endocrinology and Metabolism.

Results or Symptoms of Low Testosterone Levels.
Decreasing testosterone levels can result in:

- Loss of lean muscle
- Weight gain specially around the waistline
- Decline in libido and erectile dysfunction
- Decline in energy levels
- Irritability
- Depression, mood swings
- Decreased bone density which makes your bones more susceptible to fractures etc.

Testosterone levels in the low range (a blood serum score below 350 ng/dl) may increase your chances of dying of a heart attack. Low testosterone seems to predict increased risk of total mortality in cardiovascular disease as well as cancer," said Dr. Kay-Tee Khaw, professor of clinical gerontology at the University of Cambridge School of Clinical Medicine in Britain. There is considerable evidence of an association with depressive symptoms and low testosterone levels in men. See Amiaz, Kanayama, Pope, Seidman "Testosterone Supplementation for Depressed Men: Current Research and Suggested Treatment Guidelines" Experimental and Clinical Psychopharmacology.

How to Increase Testosterone Production Naturally.
These factors play a key role in determining and increasing testosterone levels:

1. SLEEP. Have a routine of regularly getting enough sleep. Lack of good sleep is probably the number one reason for compromised testosterone levels. Full sleep enables the body to repair and recovery. The highest release of hormones into our blood stream, including Testosterone, occurs while we sleep.

2. MAINTAIN A HEALHTY DIET AND EAT FOODS HIGH IN ZINC and MONOUNSATURATED FATS. Eating

nuritious foods in general and foots high in zinc and monounsaturated fats, in particular, raise testosterone levels. See below which foods will increase and decrease testosterone!

3. EXERCISE. Regular sustained (at least an hour) of brisk aerobic exercise three times a week will help raise your testosterone levels. Daily is better. Cycling, Hiking, walking, Swimming, Running are all good aerobic exercises to increase testosterone levels. This aerobic exercise should be at a level to increase your heart rate. Be part of a sports team!

4. LIFT WEIGHTS. Weight lifting is already known for its hormone releasing potential, but in order to really get the maximum benefit, try turning up the intensity. One way to accomplish this is by doing active recovery in between sets. You can do jump ropes, step-ups, seated balances, box jumps, jogging around the gym floor or power skips. What's important is to keep your heart rate up!

5.RECOVER FROM WORKOUTS. Recovery is an essential component of weight training and long aerobic exercise. If you overtrain -- meaning you don't allow your body to recuperate adequately between training sessions -- your circulating testosterone levels can plunge by as much as 40 percent, according to a study at the University of North Carolina.

6. COMPETE. Competition raises the sense of mission, sharpens the focus, increases metabolism and with it testosterone production.

7. KEEP ARTERIES CLEAR. The clearer the arteries, the better the body is able to deliver testosterone via the blood. Clear arteries goes a long way toward a better erection. See here for How to Naturally Maintain Clear Arteries.

8. AVOID NEGATIVE STRESS. Too much stress (negative stress as opposed to challenge)or worry depresses the immune system and reduces testosterone production.

9. HAVE CHALLENGE. Challenge and adventure, either physical, mental or emotional is a good way to get the juices flowing, including testosterone.

10. HAVE MORNING SEX. German scientists found that simply having an erection causes your circulating testosterone to rise significantly -- and having one in the morning can goose your natural post-dawn testosterone surge. Frequent sex is a good idea, is healthy and can boost testosterone. From a physiological perspective, having sex increases testosterone levels, which cause an increase in strength, energy, aggression and competitiveness. There is a big discussion about whether too frequent ejaculation is healthy in the long term. There is compelling authority that ejaculation control and discipline improves men's health, vigor, longevity and sexual vitality. See Ejaculation Frequency for Optimum Men's Health and Longevity!

11. DON'T DRINK MORE THAN 3 ALCOHOLIC DRINKS PER DAY. Alcohol affects the endocrine system, causing your testes to stop producing the male hormone.

12. DON'T SMOKE. There are studies that have shown that smoking can reduce testosterone levels and, according to a recent study by the Boston University School of Medicne, decrease genital size. In the same way that smoking has been shown to damage the ability of the blood vessels in the lungs and heart to retain elasticity, the vessels of the penis may be equally affected. The blood vessels of the penis are much smaller than those of the heart so constriction in this area may have relatively more severe consequences.

13. MANAGE WEIGHT. Obese men had a 60 percent higher chance of having a low volume of semen, according to Ghiyath Shayeb. They also had a 40 percent higher chance of having some sperm abnormalities. Ghiyath Shayeb of the University of Aberdeen presented these research results at a meeting of the European Society of Human Reproduction and Embryology.

Foods that Increase Testosterone Levels. One nutrient that should be considered absolutely essential for maintaining a man's testosterone levels is Zinc. This busy mineral is involved in almost every aspect of male reproduction, including testosterone metabolism, sperm formation, and sperm motility. Also, as medical evidence suggests that men experience a significant loss of zinc with each ejaculation, eating a food high in zinc after ejaculation is recommended.

These foods are abundant in Zinc and Vitamin B and help elevate testosterone levels naturally: Oysters not only help increase testosterone and improve libido in men but also helps increase semen production and improve sperm count, thereby giving a big boost to your fertility and potency.

Garlic is one of the the best natural ways to raise testosterone levels because it contains a strong compound called allicin that can increase the levels of testosterone hormone Other foods sources that are rich in zinc and can help enhance your testosterone levels include animal protein, Dairy and poultry products, including eggs. In fact, zinc form animal protein like Beef or red meat is more readily absorbed by your body than from any other source.

Essential fatty Acids like Omega 3 also play a key role in impacting testosterone levels positively. The best source of essential fatty acids like Omega 3 is oily fish like salmon, sardine and mackerel Nuts are good for your nuts. Research has found that men who ate diets rich in monounsaturated fat -- the kind found in peanuts -- had the highest testosterone levels. It's not known why this occurs, but some scientists believe that monounsaturated fats have a direct effect on the testes. Nuts, olive oil, canola oil and peanut butter are good sources of monounsaturated fat.

Eat cruciferous veggies. Broccoli, cauliflower and cabbage yields compounds called indoles that help lower certain estrogens, which in turn can help reduce estrogen's inhibitory effects on testosterone production.

Soy Lowers Testosterone Levels and Sperm Count, so does Refined Sugars. Eating a half serving a day of soy-based foods could be enough to significantly lower a man's sperm count, U.S. researchers have found. The study is the largest in humans to look at the relationship between semen quality and a plant form of the female sex hormone estrogen known as phytoestrogen, which is plentiful in soy-rich foods. "What we found was men that consume the highest amounts of soy foods in this study had a lower sperm concentration compared to those who did not consume soy foods," said Dr. Jorge Chavarro of the Harvard School of Public Health in Boston, whose study appears in the journal Human Reproduction. Warning! Soy has become a filler for many products, including many 'health' or 'protein' bars. Read the content labels before you buy and have your mom, wife or girlfriend read them before they buy for you. These products should be avoided by men. **Guys, the indications are that soy reduces testosterone. Why take that risk?!**

Soy, because it encourages the production of estrogen, also inhibits production of the Growth Hormone. Some Scientists also have concerns that exposure of babies to levels of phytoestrogens as high as found in infant soy formular milk is an unnecessary risk to take on behalf of the male babies. This is so because for a period after birth and lasting up to six months or more the testes are very active and levels of the male sex hormone 'testosterone' in blood can reach adult levels. Some scientists believe there is every reason to suppose that human male babies fed with soy formula milk will show a suppression of their neonatal testosterone surge.

Athletes should also note that soy protein is a rich in phytic acid which reduces mineral and trace element absorption Studies assessing markers of iron status show that supplementing isoflavone rich soy protein isolate reduces iron status by more than 7%. In contrast, the same study also showed that a whey protein supplement actually increased iron status by more than 9%. Iron is essential for oxygen transport and to maintain muscle performance, yet many athletes suffer with low iron stores. Symptoms include shortness of breath, poor exercise performance and slow recovery after exercise. It is clear that supplements containing soy proteins could bring about iron deficiency and impair exercise performance. Nutrient depleted refined carbohydrates such as refined simple sugars increase the level of insulin in blood which affects testosterone production negatively.

Unless necessary, Testosterone Supplements are Not Recommended due to potential negative side effects. Medical professionals recommend that If you have reduced levels of sexual desire, have your testosterone level checked immediately. This is so especially since low testosterone levels increase the risk of heart attack. Unless your testosterone levels are very low and need to be more quickly increased, the natural ways of increasing testosterone levels should be your first consideration. However, you can replenish your testosterone stores with injections, gels, pills or patches. Note, these medical treatments are no panacea: Side effects include acne, high cholesterol, shrunken testicles and liver damage. Further, don't take supplements like DHEA or androstenedione to boost testosterone; they might increase your risks of prostate cancer and heart disease. Ask your physician about potential side effects. There is some debate and concern whether taking Testosterone supplements decreases the ability of the body to naturally produce testosterone.

Ejaculation Frequency for Optimum Health and Longevity. The purpose of this section is to provide the differing philosophies and science upon how optimal health, testosterone levels, longevity and sexual power may be influenced by ejaculation frequency.

Eastern Philosophy on Ejaculation Frequency and Ejaculation Control. According to the eastern philosophy of Tao formulated over centuries and emphasized over and over again in Taoist literature, a man must preserve and retain his semen in order to enhance his strength, health and longevity. This philosophy believes that men that regulate their ejaculation to a minimum and retain their semen will grow strong and have a clearer mind. Furthermore, this Tao philosophy holds that men who practice ejaculation control will maintain consistently high levels of testosterone, sperm and semen and will have a stronger sexual appetite. Taoist theory believe that semen retention strengthen the brain as the essential nutrients in semen and related hormones are absorbed by the prostrate whereby they enter the blood stream and circulate throughout the body nourishing all tissues and organs, including the brain. It's a well know medical fact that semen and cerebrospinal fluids consist of the same basic incredients so preserving semen nourishes the brain by making more essential nutrients available to it.

What is the primary underlying premise behind this philosophy? Taoist thought is built upon the primary premise that every body is endowed with a limited supply of primordial energy (chee) and one's lifespan, including sexual lifespan, is determined by (i) the rate at which this energy is used up and (ii) a lifestyle that replenishes and strengthens that energy. As a bit of a man's sexual essence is used with each ejaculation, Tao teaches that ejaculation frequency should be regulated to permit a man's body to rebuild the sexual energy between ejaculations before it is used up again through ejaculation. The basic objective of Tao philosophy on ejaculation frequency is to increase as much as possible the quantity of life-giving, age-retarding hormones secreted in a man's body during sexual excitement, while at the same time decreasing as much as possible the loss of semen and its related hormones through ejaculation so that those nutrients can be reused by the body to make it stronger.

Tao Recommended Ejaculation Frequency to Increase Lifespan. "A man may attend health and longevity if he practices an ejaculation frequency of twice monthly, or 24 times a year. If at the same time he pays careful attention to proper diet and exercise, he will live a long and healthy life." Sun Simiao There are different theories among Tao theorists on how frequency should be measured. However as each man is different, we each need to determine for ourselves which level of frequency leaves us most strong and refreshed instead of tired, empty and depressed.

One Tao theorist recommends ejaculation based upon the frequency of intercourse rather than day intervals with ejaculation only 2 or 3 times in 10. The most respected of the Tao theorist, Sun Simiao, quoted above, recommends ejaculation no more than once every 20 days for men over 50 and no more than once every 100 days for men over 60. Another Tao theorist suggests ejaculation frequency should be regulated according to the seasons with recommended ejaculations (i) during spring of no more than every 3 days, (ii) twice a month in summer and fall, and (iii) not at all during the cold of winter. Another Tao theorist more recommends robust men may have more ejaculations than other men but recommends ejaculation control and restrained frequency for both. Also, as medical evidence suggests that men experience a significant loss of zinc with each ejaculation, eating a food high in zinc after ejaculation is recommended.

Tao Risks of Too Frequent Ejaculation. When sex is performed with the recommended Tao frequency, it becomes an inexhaustible source of energy, like a well that never runs dry. However, when ejaculation frequency exceeds the capacity of the body to fully replenish semen, men can experience chronic fatigue, low resistance, loss of sexual drive, loss of focus and irritability. Long term excessive ejaculation can cause chronic low zinc conditions which can cause chronic fatigue, mental confusion and significant loss of sexual drive. It is also considered harmful to ejaculate when ill, drunk or gorged with food.

Frequent Sex but Infrequent Ejaculation. Ejaculation control and discipline is not to be confused with frequency of sex. There are significant physiologic. phsycologic and therapeutic benefits to having sex. Frequent sex intercourse maintains a man's interest in the act as well as his capacity to continue indefinitely until his partner is fully satisfied.

Ejaculation Frequency and Impact on Testosterone Levels. Much of western medicine and popular culture claim that men naturally replenish their semen supply soon after ejaculation and that the male's capacity for producing semen is virtually limitless. However western and eastern athletic coaches advise their athletes to not have an ejaculation the same day prior to athletic competition as it is medically well documented that testosterone levels drop immediately after ejaculation and athletic performance is diminished.

Ejaculation Frequency and Prostate Health. Is there a correlation between ejaculation frequency and prostate health? An important consideration to men's health is whether there is any relationship between ejaculation frequency and risks to prostate cancer. Michael Leitzmann, published in the 2004 Journal of American Medical Association his research conclusions that "Our results suggest that ejaculation frequency is not related to increased risk of prostate cancer." See Ejaculation Frequency and Subsequent Risk of Prostrate Cancer. There are studies however which suggest that frequent ejaculations decreases the risk of developing prostate cancer. (See a 2008 study from the Harvard Medical School Ejaculation

Frequency and Prostate Cancer.) An issue remains whether increased ejaculations were performed by men who were healthier and as such had higher sexual activity due to better health and therefore their lower risk of prostate cancer was the result of better health due to diet and exercise and not related to ejaculation frequency.

Rates of prostate cancers vary widely across the world, with South and East Asia detecting much less frequently than in Europe, and especially the United States. This geographic disparity seems to indicate diet and lifestyle may play an important role in prostate cancer risk. As prostate cancer tends to develop in men over the age of fifty, men over fifty are encourage to regular seek medical screening regarding their prostate health.

Human Growth Hormone. The Human Growth Hormone is an important hormone for men and women that stimulates cell growth and reproduction and is an amino acid produced in the Pituitary Gland. The Pituitary Gland secretes the Growth Hormone into the blood stream for circulation to our bodies cells and organs. Our objective is to provide you information here on how to increase the natural production of the Growth Hormone for maximum health benefits and improved athletic performance. Injection of the Growth Hormone is not recommended for healthy individuals as the introduction of the artificial version may negatively impact the body's ability to naturally produce it. Injection of the artificial version is however recommended to treat natural Growth Hormone deficiency or for other medical reasons.

The Growth Hormone is important to the Longevity of everyone, but it is particularly vital to very active people and athletes. People that engage in endurance athletics like Running, Swimming and Cycling should learn what they can do to stimulate the production of this hormone.

What are the functions of the Growth Hormone? The Growth Hormone has the following vital functions:

- Increases calcium retention
- Increases mineralization of bone
- Stimulate production of bone marrow cells to produce red blood cells
- Increases protein synthesis
- Plays a role in fuel homeostasis
- Stimulates the immune system
- Increases muscle mass
- Increases the growth of all internal organs
- Promotes liver gluconeogenesis
- Promotes lipolysis

Adults deficient in the Growth Hormone have a relative decrease in muscle mass, decreased energy levels, are less vital, and have a lower quality of life. Hence the importance of living strong and healthy life, through a nutritious diet, regular vigorous exercise, and good sleep to increase the release and forestall the decline of the Growth Hormone release. The highest concentration of the Growth Hormone occurs about an hour after the first hour of sleep. Another reason why good and regular sleep is a critical factor in achieving longevity.

What Stimulates the Growth Hormone? The Growth Hormone is stimulated by:

- Sleep
- Exercise
- Low Blood Sugar Levels
- Arginine (for adults only)

There are a number of substances that increase the natural secretion of Growth Hormone. Some of them are amino acids. The most effective and economical way of causing this Growth

Hormone release appears to be taking 2 grams of the amino acid L-glutamine in the morning and taking 10 to 30 grams of the amino acid L-arginine before bedtime.

What Inhibits the Growth Hormone? The Growth Hormone is inhibited by:

- Hyperglycemia or High Blood Sugar Levels
- Exessive Estrogen
- Worry
- Lack of Sleep
- Free fatty acids

7 WOMEN'S UNIQUE HEALTH ISSUES

The purpose of this section is to (i) educate women on their unique nutritional needs and (ii) help female endurance athletes improve their health and athletic performance through optimum natural nutrition! Inadequate nutrition is common among endurance athletes in general and very common among women endurance athletes in particular. If you are a women engaged in Marathons, Ultra Running, Ironman Triathlons, competitive distance cycling or distance or open water swimming, the chances are your nutritional intake is deficient for your general health and for your peak athletic performance. All women, but in particular, women endurance athletes have unique Calcium and Iron needs and also tend to be Iron and Calcium deficient.

Key Function of Iron and the Risks of Iron Deficiency in Female Athletes. Iron is the main component of Red Blood Cells. The body contains more Red Blood Cells than any other type of cell. As each Red Blood Cell has a life span of about 120 days, Red Blood Cells must be continually replaced. On average, in every second of human life, 3 million red blood cells die and need to be replaced by 3 million new ones. Iron is essential to continually replenish Red Blood Cells. Excluding water, red blood cells are made of of about 97% Hemoglobin.

Iron is a key component of Hemoglobin which binds with oxygen molecules to deliver oxygen from the lungs to cells throughout the body.

The primary purpose of Red Blood Cells is to deliver oxygen from the lungs to cells throughout the body to generate energy. Our body's ability to delivery oxygen to the cells throughout our body efficiently as demands require determines our aerobic capacity. Maintaining a diet sufficient in natural sources of Iron is essential to produce Red Blood Cells needed to maintain optimum aerobic capacity for endurance athletes.

Women athletes of child bearing age have added need for Iron. Iron insufficiency is one of the most prevalent nutritional deficiencies among the female endurance athletes because of menstrual losses.

Iron deficiency can cause short and long term fatigue, impaired concentration and athletic performance and an impaired immune system.

Role of Calcium and Increased Need for Calcium in Women Athletes. Calcium is the most plentiful mineral in the body and plays an important role in building stronger, denser bones early in life and keeping bones strong and healthy later in life. Approximately ninety-nine percent of the body's calcium is stored in the bones and teeth.

Calcium plays other important key roles, especially important for the peak performance and health of endurance athletes, including:

- Calcium maintains strong dense bones.
- Calcium plays a key role in contraction of the heart muscle to pump blood throughout the body.
- Calcium is necessary for skeletal muscle contractions to occur.
- Calcium is essential to normal blood clotting.
- Calcium helps proper nerve impulse transmission.
- Calicum enables support of connective tissue.

Calcium deficiency in woman can lead to osteoporosis, in which the bone deteriorates and there is an increased risk of fractures. Women endurance athletes, due to the added demands for calcium that go with training and racing, have significant risks of osteoporosis caused by prolonged periods of inadequate calcium intake while training.

Vitamin K is also essential for bone formation and repair. It improves bone density and facilitates the absorption of calcium.

List of Natural Food Sources of Iron. Natural sources of Iron are preferred as they are readily utilized by the body. Iron supplement use have toxicity risks. There are two main types of Iron.

Heme Iron and Nonheme Iron. Iron is found in both animal and plant foods, but in different forms. Heme iron is derived from hemoglobin, the protein in red blood cells that delivers oxygen to cells and is found in chicken liver, oysters, clams, beef and turkey. Nonheme Iron is found in plant foods such as spinach, black eyed peas, lentils, raisans and beans and has a different chemical structure than heme Iron. Heme Iron is absorbed better than nonheme Iron. See Complete List of Natural Food Sources of Iron at Natural Sources of Iron on 1Vigor.com.

8 FOR ATHLETES (AND EVERYONE)

Ideal Performance State and Peak Performance for Athletes. The Ideal Performance State (IPS) in sports or Peak Performance for athletes is the optimal physiological and pyschological level of arousal measured by muscular tension, heart rate, blood pressure, brain wave patterns and breathing composure that results in peak performance. IPS is an important state to achieve for the endurance sports such as Running, Cycling and Swimming. IPS maximizes genetic talent. The IPS exists for every athlete. When in IPS, the athlete experiences highly distinctive patterns of feelings and thoughts which enable top performance. IPS is similar to being in the "Flow". IPS involves all levels of human existence: body, mind, emotions, spirit and creativity. IPS is reached by being in all of the following state:

* Personally challenged
* Energized with positive emotions
* Ready for fun and enjoyment
* Focused and alert
* On automatic instinct
* Relaxed and calm
* Maintaining confidence

Emotions play a key role in performance as they directly connect to arousal. Emotions are biochemical events in the brain that lead to powerful biochemical changes in the body that impact athletic performance. Empowering emotions are associated with drive, challenge, determination, persistence, fight, high energy, spirit and fun. Disempowering emotions are associated with anger, fear, temper, fatigue, helplessness, confusion, low energy. Toughness is built with the discipline of maintaining empowering emotions under the most difficult and challenging circumstance. IPS of calmness, awareness and focus create certain neurological arousal patterns within the brain. These brain patterns create a freedom that enables excellence.

The connections between emotions and internal physical chemistry are direct. One impacts the other. Diet plays such a key role in achieving IPS. Low blood sugar and low adrenaline levels are diet related and often the result of insufficient and poor quality carbohydrate intake.

Ideal Performance State for Everyone. The Ideal Performance State focused on athletic performance can be applied to everyone from the corporate executive, attorney, physician, student, parent and well, to everyone. Recently theorists have addressed the spiritual dimension—how deeper values and a sense of purpose influence performance. A successful approach to sustained high performance by everyone adopts a holistic approach that pulls together all of the Ideal Performance State elements and consider the person as a whole. Thus, an integrated theory of performance management addresses the body, the emotions, the mind, and the spirit. Jim Loehr and Tony Schwartz, The Making of a Corporate Athlete, Harvard Business Review, theorized that the same principles and skills of Ideal Performance State that have been found in top athletes can be applied to executives to help them perform at their highest potential. Although the 'Corporate Athlete' article focused upon executives, the approach can be applied to everyone in all roles of life.

High Performance Pyramid

Spiritual Capacity
Provides a powerful source of motivation, determination and endurance

Mental Capacity
Focuses physical and emotional energy on the task at hand

Emotional Capacity
Creates the internal climate that drives the Ideal Performance

State Physical Capacity
Builds endurance and promotes Mental and emotional
recovery

The premise here is that peak performance in not simply a matter of sheer brain power, but is a state of being where there is a strong and balanced spiritual, mental, emotional and physical capacity. Peak performance is achieved and maintained when the four levels are working together.

Notice that the foundation for the Ideal Performance State is physical well-being. Vigorous exercise produces a sense of emotional well-being which clears the way for peak mental performance. This higher sense of emotional well-being has a physiologically base in part resulting from the increased movement of blood throughout the body bringing nutrients and challenging the cells and organs to perform at a higher level. 1Vigor has a free online Exercise Log to help you track your exercise progress and help you stick with an exercise program.

The next building block of the Ideal Performance State is emotional Capacity. An ideal emotional state of being is one of balance. This balanced emotional state includes many positive sensations such as calmness, optimism, focus, confidence, joy, happiness and complete engagement. Negative emotions such as frustration, impatience, anger, fear, resentment and sadness tend to distract from complete engagement and can drain energy. Negative emotions can increase heart rate, blood pressure and muscle tension and otherwise create an inefficient Metabolism.

Mental Capacity is the third level of the performance pyramid. Mental capacity is enhanced through improving our cognitive capacities such as focus, Creativity Skills and Clear Thinking Skills. Focus is the ability to concentrate energy in the service of a particular productive goal. Focus skills can be improved by practicing some form of Meditation and or

Breathing composure technique. Maintaining a good diet that improves brain nutrition and includes some of the Top Ten Brain Foods plays an important role in improving Mental Capacity.

Spiritual Capacity is simply the energy that is unleashed by aligning our energy with our deepest values and lifelong productive purposes. This alignment is a powerful source of motivation. Developing Leadership Attributes can help you attain your Ideal Performance State.

Kidneys Play an Important Role in General Health and in Athletic Performance. This section is intended to provide you with (i) an appreciation of the critical role our kidneys play cleansing our blood and in the development of red blood cells, (ii) a list of nutrients, natural food sources and tips to maintain optimal kidney health, and (iii) a list of key nutrients and natural food sources needed for red blood cell production.

Having knowledge about your kidneys will help you be healthier and help athletes, especially endurance athletes (like Marathon Runners, Ironman Triathletes, Distance Cyclists and Distance Swimmers), reach peak physical performance though (i) the natural stimulation of natural EPO for the increased production of Red Blood Cells to naturally maximize our blood's oxygen carrying capacity and (ii) improved ability to keep your blood clean by filtering it of waste products. Endurance athletes, in particular, should be very focused on maintaining optimal kidney health to maximize the bodies ability to produce red blood cells, as endurance athletes tend to be slightly anemic (low blood cell count) or chronically fatigued. Studies have shown that lower hemoglobin levels (anemia) can reduce exercise capacity increasing the risk of heart failure including the risk to endurance athletes.

Each of your two kidneys are surprisingly small at about 4 to 5 inches long and about 1 inch thick, weighing in at about 4.5 to

5 ounces. Although your kidneys make up less than 0.5 percent of your total body weight, they receive close to 25 percent of the total amount of blood that your heart pumps while you're resting. Also, your kidneys use up about 20 to 25 percent of your body's supply of oxygen to support five key functions.

Five Critical Kidney Functions. The five key kidney functions are:

1. Secretion of the hormone called erythropoietin, which is responsible for stimulating the production of red blood cells in your bone marrow.

2. Keep your blood clean by filtering it of waste products and eliminating these waste products from your body as urine.

3. Help maintain your body's fluid composition.

4. Produce an enzyme called renin, which is needed to help maintain your blood pressure.

5. Convert vitamin D to its most active form.

Eastern philosophy and medicine has for centuries dwelled on the function and functional relationships of the vital organs as it relates to the vital energy at the root of life.

According to eastern medicine, the kidneys (i) store life and semen essence, (ii) house the attributes of will power, and (iii) control all sexual function, along with surrounding glands.

The Role of Kidneys in Red Blood Cell Production. Our kidney energy represents our STAMINA! In every second of human life, 3 million red blood cells die and need to be replaced by 3 million new ones. It's a complex process triggered by low oxygen levels. Our kideys play an important role in the production of red blood cells by producing a hormone called

Erythropoeitin (EPO) that initiates red blood cell production in our bone marrow, a process called Erythropoeisis. It is this hormone (EPO) that controls the rate of red blood cell production. It is interesting the the kidneys, in part, are prompted to produce EPO when the kidney detects it is receiving decreased oxygen supply. Through the stimilation of EPO, the bone marrow produces and releases into the blood stream, immature red blood cells (Reticulocytes) which mature into red blood cells within 1 to 2 days. This increased red blood cell production increases the red blood cell count in the blood thereby increasing the blood's oxygen carrying capacity.

Tips for Optimal Kidney Health. Urine that is clear and odorless is a sign of healthy functioning kidneys! Maintaining optimal kidney health helps athletes achieve peak physical performance during competition and help in the recovery process as healthier kidneys can (i) naturally produce the maximum level of EPO's necessary for the creation of Red Blood Cells to increase the bloods oxygen carrying capacity and (ii) efficiently clean the blood of waste and toxin, essential during endurance events. Stay Hydrated. Drink sufficient amounts of pure water to help your kidneys eliminate toxic chemicals and waste products. For an estimate of how much you should drink, halve your body weight and drink that in ounces of water. So, if you are 150 lbs., try to drink 75 oz. of water every day. You can exchange part of this amount with organic nonfat milk or fresh squeezed juices from organic fruits and vegetables.

If water is your primary source of hydration make sure you are taking in sufficient electrolytes. See Hydration for Endurance Athletes Natural and Nutritious Diet. Eating a natural and nutritious diet puts less stress on our kidneys blood cleansing function. The more toxins we consume in our foods, the harder our kidneys need to work to clean our blood. Two studies presented to the 2009 American Society for Nephrology have shown a relationship between diet and kidney health. One study found a link between intake of excess sodium and sweetened beverages. It's best then to avoid foods with excess salt and processed foods, which often contain excess salts. The second study found women who drank two or more servings per day of artificially sweetened soda doubled their odds of kidney function decline. Colas in particular contain high amounts of phosphoric acid, a substance known to change the urine in a way that favors kidney stone formation.

Drinking too much coffee and similar stimulants will weaken the kidneys over time. It is also believed that cold and icy foods can deplete kidney energy.

Specific Foods for Healthy Kidneys. Here is a list of foods that can help maintain healthy kidneys:

Watermelons. Occasionally Consume large quantities of Watermelons for a day, while regularly emptying your bladder. A watermelon fast.

Cranberry Juice. Pure 100% unsweetened Cranberry Juice with no additives. Cranberries are known to protect against bladder infections by preventing bacteria from sticking to the bladder wall.

Fish and Fish Oils. Studies have shown a potential beneficial role for fish and fish oil consumption in kidney health.

Egg Whites. Egg whites are pure protein and provide the highest quality of protein with all the essential amino acids. For the kidney diet, egg whites provide protein with less phosphorus than other protein sources such as egg yolk or meats.

Olive Oil. Olive oil is a great source of oleic acid, an anti-inflammatory fatty acid. The monounsaturated fat in olive oil protects against oxidation. Olive oil is rich in ployphenols and antioxidant compounds that prevent inflammation and oxidation.

Cabbage. Cabbage is packed full of phytochemicals, chemical compounds in fruit or vegetables that break up free radicals before they can do damage. High in vitamin K, vitamin C and fiber, cabbage is also a good source of vitamin B6, and folic acid. Cabbage also helps produce Testosterone.

Other Factors Impacting Kidney Health. Other things we can do to keep our kidneys health include:

The Kidney Rub and Tap. The kidney rub and tab is a brief exercise you can do to help maintain kidney health. You are able to massage your kidneys by placing the back of your hands on your skin over the location of your kidneys and rub up and down for about two to three minutes. The kidneys are located near the sides of your lower back. The kidney rub stimulates the adrenal glands and draws blood and energy to the kidneys. Tapping the same area can help dissolve crystals before they form kidney stones and stimulates the kidneys.

Maintain Low Blood Pressure. Maintaining a low blood pressure is important to kidney health as high blood pressure creates constant and significant stress on the kidneys.

Exercise. Physical exercise is another important factor to consider for optimum kidney health. Both physical activity and sweating can help your kidneys to eliminate toxins and wastes. Sedentary lifestyle contributes significantly to many health problems including obesity, heart disease, stroke, high blood pressure, diabetes, and kidney failure.

Get Enough Sleep. Good regular sleep is essential to maintain optimum kidney health.

Stress Management. Stress negatively impacts kidney function. Hot Baths or Showers When Under Stress. When under pressure and stress, hot showers or baths before bed relax tight kidneys.

Don't Eat Excessive Protein. Eating more protein than you need leads to greater workload on your kidneys, which must filter a by-product of protein metabolism called blood urea nitrogen (BUN) out of your blood. This increased workload can contribute to premature breakdown of the special capillaries (glomeruli) in your kidneys. Defining excess protein can be a bit tricky, particularly for endurance athletes with added high protein needs to aid recovery.

Don't Take Over-the-Counter Pain Pills on a Regular Basis. Non-steroidal anti-inflammatory drugs like ibuprofen (Advil, Motrin), naproxen (Aleve), and aspirin are known to cause kidney damage and disease if taken regularly. Acetaminophen (Tylenol and Excedrin) can also cause kidney damage and failure if used regularly. All of these over-the-counter pain medications probably don't pose significant danger if your kidneys are relatively healthy and you use them for emergencies only. As many professional athletes have discovered during the past several years, regular use of prescription anti-inflammatory pain medication like Vioxx, Indocin, and Naprosyn poses even greater danger to kidney health than over-the-counter pain killers.

Key Nutrients and Natural Food Sources for Red Blood Cell Production. In addition to EPO which is produced by the kidneys Iron, Vitamin B12, Folate (Vitamin B9) and Testosterone are the other key nutrients needed in the formation of Red Blood Cells. Maintaining a diet rich in these nutrients is important for endurance athletes to maintain optimum level of red blood cells to support dedicated training and peak performance during racing. A deficiency in either Iron, Vitamin B12 or Folate could cause an athlete to become slightly anemic, even chronically anemic. Iron.

Vitamin B12. Sources of Vitamin B12 include: Mollusks, clams, liver, beef, yogurt, milk, eggs, chicken. Folate. Sources of Folate include: Beef, liver, peas, pasta, spinach, asparagus, rice, broccoli, egg noodles, avocado, peanuts, wheat germ, tomato juice, orange juice, whole wheat bread, eggs, cantaloupe, papaya, and banana.

Testosterone. Page 78 has a comprehensive list of natural sources of foods that help boost testosterone.

Doping is not recommended. In the late 1980's, scientists developed and EPO like protein that, like EPO, stimulated red blood cell production. In developing this EPO like protein, these scientist were seeking to find a way to effect red blood cell production to people that were anemic (low blood cell count) due mostly to either (i) kidney disease or (ii) suppression of red blood cell production in the bone marrow caused by chemotherapy in the treatment of cancer. Athletes began to use this EPO like protein to stimulate red blood cell production to improve athlete performance through increased capacity of the blood to carry oxygen. Of course, as the main red blood cell function is to carry oxygen to cells throughout the body, the more red blood cells contained in the blood the greater will be the blood's ability to transport oxygen. Use of this EPO like protein 'Doping' has been banned by most organized athletic authorities and the use of this protein by athletes is illegal.

There are also health considerations against the use of this EPO like protein: 1. An increase in red blood cell count above normal levels increases blood viscosity or blood 'thickness' which heighten the risk of thrombotic events (strokes).

2. Regular use of this EPO like protein by athletes could disrupt the body's natural ability to produce EPO.

Mental Toughness and Mental Strength for Athletes and for Everyone.
"Pain is temporary. It may last a minute, or an hour, or a day, or a year, but eventually it will subside and something else will take its place. If I quit, however, it lasts forever." by Lance Armstrong

Mental toughness and strength is an important characteristic for athletes to acquire on the journey to reaching their Ideal Performance State and peak performance in sports. Mental Fitness is the result of mental fitness training. It is a characteristic that we all can acquire. This strength is not something that you do once, any more than you can get physically fit by one lap around the track. Mental fitness is a way of looking at your psychological health as important as your physical health.

Mental strength is having the natural or developed psychological edge that enables you to: 1. Generally cope better than your opponents with the many demands (e.g., competition, training, lifestyle) that are placed on you as a performer. 2. Specifically, to be more consistent and better than your opponents in remaining determined, focused, confident, resilient, and in control under pressure. Mental fitness training is not just for athletes to improve performance. Mental fitness training helps people cope with everyday problems and prevents these problems from overwhelming us. The resiliency that comes with mental strength is a way of thinking that allows us not to fall into self-defeating traps.

11 Characteristics of Mental Strength. Mental strength can be characterized by set of behaviors and beliefs about yourself, your objectives and how you interact with others. Here is a list of some of these behaviors:

Competitive

"The harder you work the harder it is to surrender." by Vince Lombardi

Competitors find a way to win. They take setbacks and failure to drive themselves that much harder. Competitors don't quit and refuse to loose!

Confidence

Confident athletes have a very positive can do attitude. They believe they can handle whatever comes their way.

Control

"You are really never playing an opponent. You are playing yourself." by Arthur Ashe

Successful athletes have learned to control their emotions and behavoir. Their focus is on what they can control instead of things outside of their control. Mentally tough athletes have learned the ability to maintain emotional control even under the greatest of pressure and under the most difficult of circumstances and conditions. The best athletes are in full control of their capacity and can command the control of events. Personal control is a recognition that you can't always control what happens, but you can control how you react. Mental strength comes from the realization that your success depends upon many things, but mostly depends upon you. It flows from the power and inner excellence of personal responsibility where success or failure is yours alone!

Commitment

"Everybody wants to know what I'm on. What am I on? I'm on my bike busting my ass six hours a day. What are you on?" by Lance Armstrong

"Each of us has a fire in out hearts for something. It's our goal in life to find it and keep it lit." by Mary Lou Retton

Mentally tough athletes are determined and committed to success. These athletes want to succeed more than their competitors and are willing to commit the necessary time and dedication to win.

Composure

Mental toughness requires athletes to maintain composure when the pressure is on. They have learned to maintain an ease amidst chaos.

Courage

Mentally tough athletes are willing and courage to take risks. They have the courage to push their personal limits and capabilities and push the limits reached by the winners before them.

Capacity

Strength is born in the Spiritual Capacity that provides a powerful source of motivation, determination and endurance. Deep Emotional Capacity is the heart that drives Toughness.

Concentration

"I won't even call a friend the day of a match. I'm scared of disrupting my concentration." by Chris Evert

Mentally strong athletes focus their time and enery on achieving their goals and dreams. These athlete have the concentration to develop highly focused Mental Imagery Skills. Come game day, the best athletes reach a state of highly sharp concentration to perform at their best.

Consistency

"Even if you're on the right track, you'll get run over if you just sit there." by Will Rogers

Mental strength comes from consistent training. See Running with Consistency to Run Faster by Chris Harig

Competence

Mental toughness is honing down on every detail about your sport. Lance Armstrong became as expert in natural nutritional intake for desired output and recovery. Lance drilled down on every aspect of his sport and became as good a nutritionist as he was a cyclist. Lance also sought to constantly seek ways to learn and improve his knowledge of cycling and ways to improve his performance.

Challenging

"Challenges make life interesting, however, overcoming them is what makes life meaningful." by Mark Twain Maintain

A challenging attitude!

How Mental Imagery Can Improve Skills and Athletic Performance.
"Regularly visualize yourself winning matches by running powerful, vivid and emotional images of success through your mind, seeing yourself playing brilliantly in every department of the game", by Roger Federer

Imagery can be a powerful tool for improving our skills. A bright and active imagination can facilitate progress in academic, work-related, health and social domains. This is true for many things including improving our mental capacity for playing chess, athletic performance, speech giving, and sexual performance and satisfaction. For example, mental imagery and visualization can play a key role for a new Runner finishing their first 5k or triathlon, all athletes looking to improve technique, set new personal records or finishing first.

What is Mental Imagery?   Mental imagery, also called vizualization and mental rehearsal, is the process by which we create or recreate experiences in the mind using information stored in our memory. This structured imagery is aided by a vivid imagination. The more control we have over their imagination, the more we are able to control our performance. Mental imagery is intended to train our minds and create the neural patterns in our brain to teach our muscles to do exactly what we want them to do.

Mental Imagery Enhances Skills and Athletic Performance.   Imagery has the effect of priming muscles for subsequent physical action.

Mental Imagery can have different uses in sports and in other challenges including:
1. Mental practice of specific performance skills.
2. Improving confidence and positive thinking.
3. Improving problem solving skills.
4. Controlling arousal and anxiety.
5. Preparation for performance.
6. Maintaining mental freshness during injury.

Mental Imagery Strategies.   The more clearly you are able to experience mental images and the more accurately you can control your imagined movements, the more likely you are to translate the images into superior performance. Different strategies can be employed to help implement mental imagery. Feel Movement Internally. Some like to 'feel' movement internally. This process is known as Kinaesthesis. Internally See Performance Unfold. Others like to see their performance unfold as if watching the playback from a headcam. This is known as Visual-Internal Imagery. Externally See Performance Unfold. Another frequently used type of mental imagery is referred to as Visual-External Imagery – seeing yourself perform from a distance as though watching from a grandstand or viewing video playback.

Self-Hypnosis. Self-hypnosis is a state of heightened awareness and relaxation that is self-induced where one reaches a deep state of relaxation that is extremely pleasurable. Self-hypnosis can be a valuable tool for clear mental imaging. Capturing Performance 'in the Zone'. On those rare occasions when you're performing in 'the zone' (your Ideal Performance State), it's advisable to try to 'capture in a bottle' all of the mental aspects of your performance. This will help you to recreate that optimal mindset in the future. The 4 R's.To be effective, like any skill, imagery needs to be developed and practiced regularly. There are four elements to mental imagery - Relaxation, Realism, Regularity and Reinforcement.

1. Relaxation. Having a relaxed mind and body so you can become involved in the imagery exercises. Self-hypnosis skills are helpful.

2. Realism. Create imagery so realistic you believe you are actually executing the skill. Seek clarity, vividness, emotion, control and a positive outcome!

3. Regularity. Spending between 3 and 5 minutes on imagery seems to be most effective. It should be included in training and time outside of training should be spent on imagery (10-15 minutes a day).

4. Reinforcement. Writing your imagery scripts will help you plan the content and timing of your imagery training and reinforce the image. It is possible to engage all of the above senses at once to create really vivid experiences and improve performance.

How Mental Imagery Works. Mental Imagery works in several ways to improve skills, fulfillment and athletic performance. Positive Expectations. Imagery increases our or an athlete's expectation of positive performance. This increase in expectation of positive performance consequently results in an increase in notable mental or motor performance. Building confidence also helps lower anxiety. Develops Neuromuscular Patterns. Performance involving mental motor skills are developed by strengthening and refining the connective proficiency between our brain, nervous system and muscles (neuromusclar pattern). In other words, the neural impulses passed from the brain to the muscular system during imagery may be retained in memory almost as if the movement had actually occurred.

The excitement and creation of a neuromuscular pattern associated with a particular skill can also be initiated through imagery. This connection can take place with repeated trials of imagery without the risk of physical fatigue. Thus, when we practice mental imagery, we are facilitating later physical performance. The Attention-Arousal theory on imagery suggests that the use of mental imagery helps us or athletes achieve optimal arousal level prior to a performance, task or athletic event.

How Caffeine Impacts Athletic Performance. The purpose of this section is to provide you information on (i) what is caffeine, (ii) what are the physiologic effects of caffeine (iii) how caffeine impacts athletic performance and (iv) under what circumstances and during what type of athletic events is caffeine recommended or should be avoided.

What is Caffeine? Caffeine is found in varying quantities in the beans, leaves, and fruit of some plants including the coffee plant, tea bush and kola nut. Caffeine is a physcoactive stimulant drug which primarily acts upon the central nervous system that can induce temporarily mental and physical performance, including enhanced locomotion and alertness. Caffeine is the world's most widely consumed physcoactive drug and is found in coffee, non herbal tea, manyt soft drinks and energy drinks, and is some exercise gels.

Physiologic Impacts of Caffeine. Caffeine can have the following negative impacts:

- Caffeine Inhibits Reabsorbtion of Sodium.
- Caffeine Increases Heart Rate and Blood Pressure.
- Caffeine can cause Abdominal Cramps and Diarrhea.
- Caffeine is a Diuretic. Caffeine is also a diuretic which means it can make you urinate more than usual.
- Caffeine Dehydrates. Caffeine dehydrates the body. There are some studies which indicate that caffeine does not cause dehydration and perhaps doesn't in some people. A good personal test is if caffeine causes your mouth to feel dry, then it is dehydrating you.

What is Caffeine's metabolism and half-life? Caffeine from coffee or other beverages is absorbed by the stomach and small intestine within 45 minutes of ingestion and then distributed throughout all tissues of the body. The half-life of caffeine — the time required for the body to eliminate one-half of the total amount of caffeine — varies widely among individuals, but on average, in healthy adults, caffeine's half-life is approximately 4.9 hours. Caffeine readily crosses the blood-brain barrier that separates the bloodstream from the interior of the brain. Once in the brain, the principal mode of action is as an antagoinist of andenosine receptors. The caffeine molecule is structurally similar to andenosine , and binds to adenosine receptors on the surface of cells.. Therefore, caffeine acts as a competitive inhibitor. Adenosine is found in every part of the body, because it plays a role in the fundamental ATP-related energy metabolism.

So how does caffeine impacts athletic performance? High levels of caffeine use, such as 800 mg per day, have been banned by the International Olympic Committee and other institutions. Some athletes have come close to flunking the drug test after ingesting only 350mg. Caffeine can cover up the fact that your body needs more rest. Rest is essential to peak athletic performance. Caffeine effects each person differently. Some people feel like they have more energy and can exercise harder and longer if they have caffeine first. Caffeine makes other people feel too jittery or nervous to do well during sports activities. It may not be good for you to take caffeine if you are nervous or get pre-event jitters.

Caffeine can make you more nervous, cause muscle shakiness, and make it hard to concentrate. Studies have shown that caffeine helped muscles use fat as a fuel, sparing the glycogen stored in muscles and increasing endurance. But there were several hints that something else was going on. For example, caffeine improved performance even in short intense bursts of exercise when endurance is not an issue. Some researchers report that caffeine increases the power output of muscles by releasing calcium that is stored in muscle. Athletes may also experience abdominal cramps and diarrhea related to the large intestine contractions caused by caffeine. The combination of dehydration and cramping can have particularly detrimental effects on performance. Don't over use caffeine prior to and during a race. Terry Graham, chairman of the Department of Human Health and Nutritional Sciences of the University of Guelph in Canada, found that at 9 milligrams per kilogram, athletes actually did worse.

Caffeine Quantity in Sports Drinks and Sports Supplements. How do I know how much caffeine is right for me? Ask your caregiver before using caffeine to improve your ability to do sports. If you do not usually drink coffee or other things with caffeine, Try 50 to 100 mg of caffeine at first. The highest amount that most people can tolerate before hard exercise is 350 mg. Another way to figure the best amount of caffeine for you is to take it according to how much you weigh. Take 2 to 4 mg of caffeine for each kilogram (kg) of your body weight. Divide your weight in pounds by 2.2 to figure out how much you weigh in kilograms. For example, a 154 pound athlete weighs 70 kilograms and could take 140 to 320 mg of caffeine. Caffeine is readily available in a variety of products:

Gu, Vanilla, 1 oz: 20 mg
Diet Coke, 12 oz: 30 mg
Espresso, 5 oz shot: 150 mg
Brewed Coffee, 8 oz: 150 mg
Jolt gum, 1 piece: 40 mg
Pepsi, 12 oz can: 45 mg
Dexatrim diet pill: 52 mg
Excedrine, 1 tab: 5 mg
NoDoz max, 1 tab: 200 mg
Starbucks, 16 oz: 200 mg
Red Bull, 8 oz can: 80 mg
Chocolate milk, 8 oz glass: 10 mg
Semi-sweet chocolate, 1 oz: 20 mg
Black tea brewed 3 minutes, 6 oz: 50 mg

Developing a Caffeine Strategy for Peak Athletic Performance. Many athletes and coaches are not caffeine fans. There are many studies which show caffeine enhances athletic performance. On the flip site, researchers in Switzerland advise athletes to refrain from consuming caffeine prior to races, as they have found caffeine limits the body's ability to increase blood flow to the heart, which is needed to deliver increased oxygen needs during exercise. Despite some known benefits of caffeine in some exercise, individual results may vary greatly. Differences in metabolism, diet, and frequency of caffeine use are some of the factors that can determine how an individual will react to caffeine. Additionally, some athletes may actually experience a decrease in performance, usually due to side effects of caffeine. Sprints. Research has shown that pre-exercise caffeine enhances performance in sprints, short distances events, and in all-out efforts lasting four to five minutes.

Here are a few tips for using caffeine:

1. Endurance Events and Ironman Triathlons. Because longer races like Marathons and Ironman Triathlons have a greater baseline risk of dehydration, nausea and abdominal cramps, it is very important to consider the side effects of caffeine use during these distance events. As there inevitably is a down associated with the initial up provided by caffeine, endurance athletes will want to become familiar with how caffeine affects them during competition to lessen the risk of bonking during the later stages of a race.

2. No Caffeine One Week Prior to Race. Caffeine only aids the performance of athletes who do not habitually use caffeine. So if you are a regular coffee drinker and want to benefit from a caffeine boost, you need to cut out the caffeine for two weeks before a big race.

3. Moderate Dose. Have a moderate dose between 1-2 hours prior to your race prior to short course races.

4. Familiarity. Make sure that you have used caffeine under a variety of training conditions and are thoroughly familiar with how your body reacts to this drug. Never try anything new on race day.

5. Weather Conditions. If weather conditions exist which can cause severe dehydration, such as very windy, humid, hot or cold, use of caffeine because of its dehydrating effects should be very limited, particularly for endurance events.

6. Recovery. Caffeinated drinks or supplements are not recommended when rapid rehydration after exercise is desired because caffeine can promote modest diuresis in some individuals.

Rest and Recovery. Rest and recovery builds high energy levels for everyone, especially athletes. Good management of our rest and recovery helps us maintain a high energy level and a high and efficient metabolism. Effective energy management has two key components. The first is the rhythmic movement between energy expenditure, which can also be called stress, and energy renewal which occurs during recovery. In the arena of sports, we have learned that the real enemy of high performance is not stress, which is actually the stimulus for growth. Rather, the problem is the absence of disciplined recovery. Chronic stress without recovery depletes energy reserves, leads to burnout and breakdown, and ultimately undermines performance. Routines that promote the cycle of stress and recovery build athletic skills.

Hydration and Endurance Athletes. The purpose of this section is to (i) educate you on the physiologic role hydration plays in endurance athletic performance and injury prevention, (iii) have you learn the warning signs of dehydration, (iv) teach the importance of maintaining electrolyte balance when considering hydration, (v) recommend specific hydration quantity, (vi) suggest the benefits of nonfat milk as a healthy hydration source and (vii) help you be a better athlete!

What is the Function of Hydration? Our body composition is 66% water. Fluid and electrolyte balance is a major function of homeostasis, which is our body's ability to maintain its internal environment as it adjusts to challenges and stress. To the extent our bodies are able to adjust to these challenges the state of good health is maintained. Proper hydration is important for cellular metabolism, blood flow and therefore athletic performance.

Warning Signs of Dehydration

If your are feeling thirsty, you are already somewhat dehydrated. The warning signs of dehydration include:

- Thirst
- Muscle cramping
- Headaches
- Dry mouth
- Weakness
- Unclear thinking
- Fatigue
- Bloating
- Dark yellow urine
- Significant weight loss during exercise
- Decrease of sweat during exercise

Fluid Intake Requirements for Distance Runners, Cyclists, Hikers, Swimmers and Ironman Triathletes

The best hydration strategy for endurance runners, cyclists, swimmers and Ironman triathletes is to maintain focus on staying fully hydrated beginning one week before race day. **Good hydration is especially critical for the two to three days prior to race day.**

To determine how much water you should be consuming on a daily basis, divide your body weight by half. That is amount of water in ounces you should be consuming daily without exercise. Add another 8 to 16 ounces for every 60 minutes of exercise you do.

Cyclists are recommended to drink 24oz of fluid each hour cycling for distance events.

Runners are recommended to drink 16- 27oz of fluid each hour running for distance events.

The amount of fluid intake will be greatly impacted by weather conditions.

Another measure of adequate fluid intake is body weight. Athletes are recommended to weigh themselves daily prior to training so they can become aware of decreases in body weight due to dehydration. Athletes who are down 1-2% in body weight can be assumed to be dehydrated.

Note, that too much fluid can cause GI distress. The speed at which a beverage travels from the stomach in to the small intestine (the gastric emptying rate) depends on the energy content (calories) and volume of the beverage consumed. A small concentration of carbohydrate will encourage rapid absorption, but too much carbohydrate will slow gastric emptying and can result in GI distress.

Hydration and Electrolyte Balance. Maintaining Hydration and Electrolyte Balance is critical to nerve and muscle function, and as such, is a key consideration for athletes hoping to achieve their optimum athletic performance. Electrolytes are molecules capable of conducting eletrical impulses and include sodium, potassium, calcium, magnesium, and chloride. **Both muscle tissue and neurons are considered electric tissues of the body. Muscles and neurons are activated by electrolyte activity!**

Muscle contraction is dependent upon the presence of calcium (Ca^{2+}), sodium (Na^+), and potassium (K^+). Without sufficient levels of these key electrolytes, muscle weakness or severe muscle contractions may occur.

Hyponatremia, a low concentration of sodium in the blood, has become more prevalent in ultra-endurance athletes. The Hawaii Ironman Triathlon routinely sees finishers with low blood sodium concentrations. Adequate sodium balance is necessary for transmitting nerve impulses and proper muscle function, and even a slight depletion of this concentration can cause problems. Ultra distance running events that take place in hot, humid conditions, and have athletes competing at high intensity have conditions prime for hyponatremia to develop.

During high intensity exercise, sodium is lost along with sweat. **An athlete who only replaces the lost fluid with water may contribute to a decreased blood sodium concentration.** Fluids with electrolytes are recommended for athletes during performance, especially during endurance events. It's also advisable to carry salt pills on a race. It's a good idea to take a salt pill (with water) at the start of specific muscle pain.

Hydration Needs of Runners, Hikers and Cyclists in Hot, Humid, Windy or Cold Weather. Once the body starts to become dehydrated, it can't function at its full capacity and as normal metabolism becomes impaired, your health and athletic performance is at risk. Dehydration risks increase during hot, humid, windy and cold weather.

Cold Weather Hydration. Surprisingly, dehydration is also a winter hazard. Sweat may not pour from your brow the way it does in summer, but depending on your level of exertion and the dryness of the air, significant moisture loss occurs. Also, fluid intake normally drops because people don't crave cold drinks during the winter.

The onset of dehydration often times is the cause of hypothermia. Hypothermia is very possible during endurance training and competitions (like Marathons and Ironman Triathlons) conducted in the cold. A person can become hypothermic if the rate of heat production during exercise is exceeded by the rate of heat loss. Dehydration and then Hypothermia causes a lower cellular metabolic rate which further decreases body temperature. During hypothermia blood volume decreases due to inadequate fluid intake reducing central nervous system and key organ functions.

Mountaineers are well aware drinking plenty of fluids during cold weather is essential to maintain core body temperatures to safely tackle the mountains in winter. Runners and cyclists should become equally aware of this need when training and racing in cold conditions.

Hot Weather Hydration. The debilitating effects of heat stress on the ability to perform prolonged strenuous exercise are well established. During exercise in a hot environment, a substantial rise in body core temperature is often linked with the onset of fatigue. Fluid replacement before and during prolonged exercise in the heat has been shown to be effective in reducing the elevation of body temperature and in extending endurance capacity.

Recent studies have show that **ingestion of a cold drink before and during exercise in the heat reduced physiological strain** (reduced heat accumulation) during exercise, leading to an improved endurance capacity. **Exercise time was longer with the cold drink than with the warm drink, as the cold drink lowered heart rate, lowered skin and core temperature**. Drinking cold drinks during exercise also reduced the need to sweat, resulting in a longer sweating capacity.

When exercising in hot weather, the combination of the external heat and the internal heat produced from the exercise, heat within the body can build causing Hyperthermia which is having a core body temperature that is too high.

Maintaining good hydration can reduce the onset of Hyperthermia as good hydration enhances sweating which acts to cool core body temperatures.

Scientific data supports the position that **caffeine reduces heat tolerance** during exercise in a hot environment, via three physiological mechanisms. First, the diuretic effect of caffeine may exaggerate the declines that occur with plasma volume and stroke volume. Second, caffeine stimulates the sympathetic nervous system, and it may increase sweat rate. Third, caffeine increases resting metabolic rate in physically trained and sedentary individuals; this may increase heat storage and internal body temperature. These effects reduce heat tolerance (i.e., the exercise time to fatigue or exhaustion) by exacerbating dehydration and increasing body temperature.

Humid Weather Hydration. In very humid weather, our sweat doesn't evaporate as very well and we tend to sweat more with less cooling effect thereby loosing needed fluids to maintain good performance. Fatigue will begin to increase when fluids are not replaced and under extreme lack of fluid replacement heat exhaustion or stroke can occur.

Wind Caused Dehydration. Windy conditions whether hot or cold can sap moisture from your body even when standing still. Extra hydration is necessary during windy conditions.

Acclimate. When training or racing in weather conditions very different from your training environment, it is recommendedl to arrive at the venue 4 days prior to the event, to enable the body to adjust to the different environment to reach a hydration balance consistent with this new environment.

Benefits of Nonfat Milk for Hydration. Milk is an excellent primary source of hydration as it is composed of 87% water and 13% solids. Milk solids are composed of 37% Lactose (a carbohydrate), 27% Protein, 30% Fat and 6% Minerals. Milk Protein consists of 20% Whey and 80% Casein. Milk also is an excellent source of calcium (to build strong bones and muscle), protein, carbohydrates and Vitamin D.

Milk also contains just the right percentage of potassium and sodium that supports maximum nutrient absorption and helps maintain ideal electrolyte balances. Nonfat milk or low fat milk is preferred in the warm climates and during summer. Low fat milk or whole milk is better in the winter as the extra natural fats help generate heat internally to stay warm. Whole milk is also better for younger athletes as the younger athletes needs the added fats to maintain their higher metabolism. Milk, especially non or low fat, may be a better hydration source than relying primarily on water. Milk is also good food.

The bottom line, milk contains all the hydration and nutrients to fuel endurance training and competition. . . . and its natural!

Hydration and Recovery. Immediately after prolonged training or events, athletes can be dehydrated, mildly hypoglycemic (lower than normal blood glucose levels) and have low electrolyte levels. Low blood glucose levels can be dangerous as glucose is the primary source of fuel to the brain. Good hydration within 45 minutes of endurance training or event is essential to aid recovery. Fluids along with protein and carbohydrates soon after an endurance event will help avoid post race injury and help to repair and rebuild damaged tissue. It is important very soon after prolonged exercise that blood, liver and muscle glycogen levels be replenished. A sports recovery drink with carbohydrates and electrolytes is recommended. Whole, nonfat or chocolate milk is also an excellent recovery drink.

How to Recover from Endurance Events. Developing an effective recovery strategy is essential to peak performance and injury prevention. Fatigue and energy depletion occurs after Ironman Triathlons, Marathons, Ultras and other endurance sport training and events, long bike rides, climbing, hikes, or after long periods of physical activity. Although endurance athletes have acute recovery needs, developing a recovery strategy and overcoming fatigue is important to all athletics and the physically active.

This fatigue has several causes including:
(i) low liver and intramuscular glycogen levels, and low blood glucose levels,
(ii) muscle tissue damage that decreases the contractile and elasticity ability of the muscle,
(iii) neural and central nervous system fatigue, in part caused by electrolytes depletion, that impairs neuromuscular function,
(iv) lower levels of testosterone and the growth hormones (HGH and IGF-1) which are needed for physiolgic and psychological recovery.

11 Recover Stratecies. To quicken and aid recovery it is recommended:

1. Rehydrate. Rehydration is mission critical. Begin hydration immediately after your training or event and continue hydrating until your pretraining or event weight is obtained.

2. Restore Healthy Glycogen and Glycose Levels. Beginning within 20 minutes after a long workout, have small meals of carbohydrates every 30 minutes for 3 hours, to restore glycogen and glucose to healthy levels.

3. Restore Electrolyte Balance. Electrolyte rebalance should begin immediately by consuming natural sources of electrolytes such as milk and bananas. For a list of natural sources of electrolytes

4. Lower Resting Heart Rate. Lowering your resting heart rate is important to quicken your recovery!

5. Amino Acid and Protein Intake. Amino acid and protein uptake is three times fasster and greater than normal after a good workout. Milk, yogurt, or a tuna fish sandwich are good quick protein sources.

6. Naturally Encourage Production of Testosterone and the Growth Hormone. Testosterone and the growth hormones development are enhanced during sleep and rest, and suppressed during stress, including the stress of endurance events. A nap within a few hours of activity will increase hormone development essential to rebuilding muscle and recovery.

7. Replenish Nutrients for Natural Red Blood Cell Production. Red blood cell production begins when the kidneys detect low blood oxygen levels. When blood oxygen levels are low, the kidneys produce Erythropoietin, a hormone which starts the formation of red blood cell production. Red blood cell production then relies upon an adequate supply of Iron, Vitamin B12, Folate and Testosterone. After an endurance event, the body needs these nutrients to produce new red blood cells essential to prevent fatigue and deliver adequage oxygen to the cells.

8. Reduce Infammation. There are several ways to reduce inflammation including (i) icing (ii) compression garments, (iii) elevation, (iv) massage, (v) stretching, and (vi) hydrostatic pressure, where the weight of water (eg. ice baths) reduces inflammation.

9. Sleep, Rest and Relax. Sleep, rest and relaxation are essential to recovery.

10. Active Recovery.. Taking an easy short walk, run, swim, hike, or bike ride is a good way to encourage recovery.

11. Cool Down. Perform a 15 minute cool down at very low intensity immediately after long activity.

9 LIFESTYLE AND PHILOSOPHY

Lifestyle Simplicity Enhances Life Quality and Longevity.
Plato used the expression techne tou biou which means 'the craft of life' and refers to the art of crafting and shaping life. Modern culture and excess stress has (i) caused many to loose control over their life, (ii) dulled peoples skills and ability to craft their life mission, and (iii) dampened the spirits of many. Loss of control and dampened spirits can cause depression. Also, two new studies firmly establish anxiety as an independent predictor for subsequent coronary heart disease years down the line.

Crafting a simple lifestyle helps people gain control over their life and is a recipe for good, long, quality living. Lifestyle simplicity offers a practicle down-to-earth philosophy of life that values caring for the soul or spirit. Lifestyle simplicity helps us achieve our goals and reach an inner harmony, peace and a state of grace. A simple lifestyle does not at all mean a boring or dull life or a life of little quantity or accomplishment. Note though that quantity will not make up for a lack of quality. Nor is a simple life a perfect life. It might turn out the more simple one's lifestyle, the more we may accomplish. A simple lifestyle is having a singleness of eye in achieving one's life mission and goals. Lifestyle simplicity is achieved through (i) caring for the spirit and soul (ii) establishing worthy lifetime missions, (ii) setting priorities to work toward those missions (iii) regular genuine rest, (iv) humbleness, and (v) development of appreciation for the simple pleasures.

Care of the Spirit. When life becomes too busy we usually don't take the time to nourish our soul and spirit. But first, what is our soul or spirit? Soul or spirit is not a thing, but a quality or a dimension of experiencing life and ourselves. It has a lot to do with depth, value, relatedness, heart, and personal substance. It also has a lot to do with self-knowledge and self-acceptance which is possible after we come in tune with our being, needs and nature. Cultivation and care of our spirit takes time, effort and some skill. It's like a lifelong husbanding of raw materials like the farmers who cultivates their fields to produce excellent crops.

Care of the spirit starts first with a humble approach that accepts our human foibles. Care of our soul is a process that concerns itself not so much with 'fixing' a central flaw as with attending to the small details of everyday life, as well as to major changes and decisions. However, the spiritually disturbing feelings of envy and jealousy are not to be left raw wallowing in them for long periods of time. Our goal is not to make life problem-free, but to give ordinary life the depth and value that comes with cultivating our spirit. The result is a richly elaborated life connected to our important relationships, society and nature. Care of the soul requires that we sustain the experiences of absence, wandering, longing, melancholy, separation, chaos and deep adventure. Fulfilling work, rewarding relationships, personal power and relief from symptoms of distress are all gifts from the soul . . . . from the soul that has been well cared for!

Power of the Soul. In the soul, power doesn't work the same way as it does in the ego and will, where we garner our strength, develop a strategy and apply every effort. The power of the soul, in contrast, is more like a great reservoir and more like the force of water in a fast moving river. The power of the soul is natural, not manipulated, and seemingly stems from from an unknown source. A powerful soul enriches our love of life.

Tips to a Simple Life.
"What lies behind us and what lies before us are tiny matters compared to what lies within us." Oliver Wendell Holmes

It is our artful task to find artful means for articulating and structuring the power of the soul and to thrust this power into life for the purpose of achieving our missions and life goals. Here's a good exercise to help you develop your missions and lifetime goals. Imagine yourself going to a funeral for a loved one. As you walk to the front of the room and look inside the casket, you suddenly come face to face with yourself. This is your funeral three years from now. As you look around the room to the people attending your service, what would you like each of the speakers to say about you and your life? Think deeply! What kind of husband, wife, father or mother would you like their words to reflect? What type of son or daughter? What kind of friend? What kind of work associate. What kind of community member? What type of character, contributions, achievements would you like them to remember? Now, establish your missions and life goals! Set priorities and maintain a simple lifestyle to accomplish this dream.

Securing Genuine Rest and Rejuvenation plays a big role in quality living. When we become to busy often we do not achieve genuine rest and may forget how to achieve genuine rest. Genuine rest is achievable through a simple lifestyle. The rhythmn of work and rest is the natural order nature and in the human condition. Rest is at the base of healthy living. Rest gives us an opportunity to fill our private world with vigor and joy. Meaning and Purpose of Genuine Rest. The meaning and purpose of genuine rest is to help us maintain order in our private worlds. This rest in not a luxury, but rather a necessity for those who want good health, growth and maturity.

Genuine Rest. Genuine rest is the cessation of the routine of our lives. Rest is not leisure or amusement, as leisure and amusement do not provide order to our lives. Fun filled moments, diversion, laughter, recreation, leisure and amusement are necessary, but they alone will not restore the soul as genuine rest. Genuine rest penetrates to the deepest levels of fatique in our inner world so that we can be physically and spiritually renewed and rejuvenated. Genuine rest is a time of looking backward and of closing the loop to survey what has been accomplished by our work. Rest is a necessary exercise for the appreciation and dedication of our routines. Rest is meant first and foremost to provide us an opportunity to (i) interpret our work and relationships, (ii) give meaning to our work and relationships, and (iii) make sure we know whom or for what it is properly dedicated. Rest helps us sort out the truth and commitments by which we live. Rest keeps us on course to achieve our Missions.

Tools to help Achieve Genuine Rest. There are a few questions we can ask ourselves to help us achieve genuine rest and provide meaning to our lives relationships and work:

1. What does my work mean?
2. For whom did I do this work?
3. How well was the work done?
4. Why did I do this?
5. What results did I expect?
6. What did I receive?
7. How and why is a particular relationship important?
8. How has a relationship been improved?
9. How does my work and relationships relate to the larger community?

We need to take time from our busy and frantic pace to take inventory of the significance of our work, relationships and the purpose and mission of our life. The person who establishes a block of time for genuine rest on a regular basis is more than likely to keep all of life in proper perspective and remain free from burnout and breakdown.

Use of Time. The essence of the best thinking in the area of time management can be captured in a single phrase: Organize and execute around priorities. There are important questions to ask yourself regarding the use of your time. Take time for that purpose as it is a valuable inquiry. Follow-up periodically with the same inquiry. Then, establish your priorities so that your missions are accomplished. How are you allocating sufficient time with to reflect to achieving your Mission? How are you allocating your time for the purpose of personal growth and service to others? Are you taking the time to meditate and reflect upon your actions over the past week. What are you doing with your mind and though process? Are you allocating your responsibilities and 'project's to enable genuine rest. Some people find unique solitude and quiet while running, cycling, hiking, swimming and climbing. Typically these athletes have reached a relative level of proficiency and skill that they are able to participate in their sport and yet find the quiet space for quality reflection. Some find the quiet time to meditate through prayer. Other's have developed mediation skills through the mental and physical disciplines such as Yoga or Qigong. While others find this peace while taking long walks.

Leadership.   Leadership or followership experience impacts longevity and fullness of life. If we can make our experiences with those companions fulfilling, certainly our lives will be fuller and more vigorous. The word "fulfilling" is intended to acknowledge that it is unrealistic to assume pain free or loss free leadership or followership experience. Instead the manner in which we as leaders and followers transit difficulties and move on has substantial bearing on short and long term success. Successful leadership also has the potential to enhance individual longevity. For an interesting discussion on how Leadership contributes to life quality and lifespan, see *Leadership Contributes to a Vigorous Life* by Dan Ballbach on 1Vigor.com .

ADDITIONAL RECOMMENDED READING

The following books and publications are recommended to the reader for additional general background and specific information on the various topics covered in this book. This list is a partial bibliography of the materials used in researching Natural Health - Peak Performance - Longevity Lifestyle.

Books

Food for Fitness, Chris Carmichael
The Art of Happiness, Dalai Lama
The Tao of Health, Sex and Longevity, Daniel Reid
The Complete Book of Chinese Health and Healing,
    Daniel Reid
Power Aging, Gary Null
Mind Gym, Gary Mack
The Brain Trust Program, Larry McLeary
Multiple Intelligences, Howard Gardner
Exercise Physiology, George Brooks
The New Toughness Training for Sports, James Loehr
Building Powerful Nerve Force, Paul Bragg
The Purpose Driven Life, Rick Warren
The 7 Habits of Highly Effective People, Steven Covey
Total Immersion, Terry Laughlin
Care of the Soul, Thomas Moore
Pulling Your Own Strings, Wayne Dyer
Loneliness: Human Nature and the Need for Social Connection, John
    Cacioppo
*Coaches' Guide to Enhancing Recovery in Athletes: A
    Multidimensional Approach to Developing a "Performance
    Lifestyle"*, Ian Jeffreys
*The Omega-3 Connection: The Groundbreaking Antidepression Diet
    and Brain Program*, Andrew Stoll
The Natural Testosterone Plan: For Sexual Health and Energy,
    Stephen Harrad Buhner

*Practicing the Power of Now: Essential Teachings, Meditations, and
Exercises from the Power of Now,* Eckhart Tolle
Psychology of Intelligence Analysis, Richards J. Heuer, Jr.,
Central Intelligence Agency
Quick Thinking on Your Feet: The Art of Thinking Under Pressure,
Valerie Pierce

Publications

Vitamin D Metabolism, Bodo Lehmann, Carl Gustov Carus
Medical School, Dresden University of Technology,
Dresden, Germany, Dermatologic Therapy 2010
Vitamin D and Innate Immunity, Jeremiah Miller, Departments
of Medicine, University of California at San Diego,
Dermatologic Therapy 2010
Health Effects of Vitamin D, Heike Bischoff-Ferrari,
University of Zurich, Switzerland, Dermatologic Therapy
2010
Photoprotection: a Review of the Current and Future Technologies,
Steven Wang, Memorial-Sloan-Kettering Cancer Center,
Dermatologic Therapy 2010
*Effects of Ambient Sunlight and Photoprotection on Vitamin D
Status,* Joseph Diehl, Departments of Medicine at UCLA,
Dermatologic Therapy 2010
*Low Prenatal Sunlight Exposure May Increase Multiple Sclerosis
Risk,* Pauline Anderson and Laurie Barclay, MD,
Medscape
Low Testosterone Linked to Increase Risk of Death, Professor
Kay-Tee Khaw, University of Cambridge School of
Clinical Medicine
Soy Formula Can Reduce Testosterone Levels, Dr. Richard
Sharpe, Medical Research Council Human Reproductive
Sciences Unit in Edinburgh
Soy Based Foods May Lower Sperm Count, Julie Steenhuysen,
Reuters

Men With High Testosterone May Live Longer, Metaba.Net

Effect of Exercise on Serum Sex Hormones in Men: A 12- Month Randomized Clinical Trial , Vivian N. Hawkins, Medicine and Science in Sports and Exercise

Soy Linked to Low Sperm Count, HealthDay News

Physiological, Cognitive and Psychological Benefits of Yoga by Christina Geithner, 1Vigor.com

Depression Basics, Everyday Health

Implications of Marked Weight Gain Associated With Antipsychotic Medications in Children and Adolescents, Christopher K. Varley, MD, JAMA

Smoking and Mental Illness: Results From Population Surveys in Australia and the United States, David Lawrence, BMC Public Health

Antidepressants Linked to Increased Risk for Death, Stroke in Postmenopausal Women , Pam Harrison, Medscape Medical News

Antidepressants May Only Be Effective in Treatment of the Severest Depression, Caroline Cassels, Medscape Medical News

Whole Diet May Ward Off Depression and Anxiety, Caroline Cassels, Medscape Medical News

Unintentional Drug Poisoning (overdose) Deaths: A National Epidemic , Bret Stetka, MD, Medscape

Broad Review of FDA Trials Suggests Antidepressants Only Marginally Better than Placebo, Deborah Brauser, Medscape

Sports Massage Helps Performance, Jessica Ippoliti, 1Vigor.com

The Making of a Corporate Athlete, Jim Loehr and Tony Schwartz, Harvard Business Review

What is Mental Toughness and How to Develop It?, David Yukelson, Ph.D., Penn State University

Combined Impact of Health Behaviors and Mortality in Men and Women, Professor Kay-Tee Khaw, University of Cambridge School of Clinical Medicine

Anxiety Predicts Heart Disease Years Later, Lisa Nainggolan, Heartwire, Medscape

A Theory of Human Motivation, A. H. Maslow, York University

The Human Hierarchy of Needs, Turil Cronburg

Nutrient Effects on the Nervous System, Eric H. Chundler, University of Washington

Clear Thinking: Creating a Longer More Productive Life, Valerie Pierce, 1Vigor.com

Aerobic Exercise and Creative Potential: Immediate and Residual Effects, David M. Blanchette, Creativity Research Journal

Critical Thinking: What It Is and Why It Counts, Dr. Peter A. Facione

Valuable Intellectual Traits, Richard Paul and Linda Elder

Leadership Contributes to a Vigorous Life, Dan Ballbach, 1Vigor.com

Running with Consistency to Run Faster, Chris Harig, 1Vigor.com

Ultrarunning Hydration, James Styler, 1Vigor.com

Hydration and Electrolytes -Impact on Athletic Performance, by Paul B. Bennett, Jr., 1Vigor.com

ABOUT THE AUTHOR

Ralph Teller has been a student of Longevity since his studies at Fordham University where he earned his B.A. Ralph founded 1Vigor.com focused on natural health, peak performance and longevity. Ralph is also an Ironman Triathlete and is a Finisher at the 2004 Ironman California 70.3, 2005 Ironman Canada, 2006 Ironman UK, 2007 Ironman (Germany) European Championship, 2008 Lake Stevens Ironman 70.3, 2008 Longhorn Ironman 70.3, 2009 Ironman Boise 70.3, and 2010 Ironman Calgary 70.3. A Basic Climb graduate from the Mountaineers, he has hiked and climbed many of the peaks in Washington State, including Mount Rainier. A lawyer in Washington State, he received his J.D. from Gonzaga University Law School, and was General Counsel to Shurgard and helped the company establish a national footprint. Ralph was also VP Business Development & General Counsel to software developer Raima Corporation where he played a key role in quadrupling revenues over 17 consecutive profitable quarters that resulted in a successful acquisition by a publicly traded company. Ralph is the father of two children, and has lived in Fall City, Washington the past 20 years. Email Ralph: ralph@1vigor.com